AGELESS

INTENSITY

HIGH-INTENSITY WORKOUTS TO SLOW THE AGING PROCESS

Pete McCall, CSCS

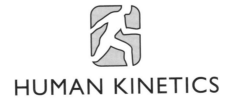

HUMAN KINETICS

Library of Congress Cataloging-in-Publication Data

Names: McCall, Pete, 1972- author.
Title: Ageless intensity : high-intensity workouts to slow the aging
  process / Pete McCall.
Description: Champaign, IL : Human Kinetics, 2022. | Includes
  bibliographical references.
Identifiers: LCCN 2021003224 (print) | LCCN 2021003225 (ebook) | ISBN
  9781718200753 (paperback) | ISBN 9781718200760 (epub) | ISBN
  9781718200777 (pdf)
Subjects: LCSH: Physical fitness for older people. | Exercise for older
  people.
Classification: LCC GV482.6 .M33 2022 (print) | LCC GV482.6 (ebook) | DDC
  613.7/0446--dc23
LC record available at https://lccn.loc.gov/2021003224
LC ebook record available at https://lccn.loc.gov/2021003225

ISBN: 978-1-7182-0075-3 (print)

Senior Acquisitions Editor: Michelle Maloney; **Managing Editor:** Hannah Werner; **Copyeditor:** Christina Nichols; **Permissions Manager:** Dalene Reeder; **Senior Graphic Designer:** Sean Roosevelt; **Cover Designer:** Keri Evans; **Cover Design Specialist:** Susan Rothermel Allen; **Photograph (cover):** Cavan Images / Getty Images; **Photographs (interior):** Nicholas Pappagallo, Jr., photos in chapters 3 and 4 and on p. 189; Graham Koffler, photos in chapter 6 and on pp. 11, 179, 205, 207, and 209; All other photos © Human Kinetics, unless otherwise noted; **Photo Asset Manager:** Laura Fitch; **Photo Production Manager:** Jason Allen; **Senior Art Manager:** Kelly Hendren; **Illustrations:** © Human Kinetics, unless otherwise noted; **Printer:** Premier Print Group

We thank the Parkwood Photography Studio in Phoenix, Arizona, and Core Health & Fitness in Lake Forest, California, for assistance in providing the locations for the photo shoots for this book.

Human Kinetics books are available at special discounts for bulk purchase. Special editions or book excerpts can also be created to specification. For details, contact the Special Sales Manager at Human Kinetics.

Printed in the United States of America   10 9 8 7 6 5 4 3 2 1

Human Kinetics
1607 N. Market Street
Champaign, IL 61820
USA

United States and International
Website: **US.HumanKinetics.com**
Email: info@hkusa.com
Phone: 1-800-747-4457

Canada
Website: **Canada.HumanKinetics.com**
Email: info@hkcanada.com

E8200

Tell us what you think!
Human Kinetics would love to hear what we can do to improve the customer experience. Use this QR code to take our brief survey.

This book is dedicated to the loves of my life, Parker and Ryan, my daughters. They inspire me to be active every day so that we can spend time together for many, many years to come.

Contents

Exercise Finder

*This exercise includes one or more variations.

Foreword

I have to admit that I haven't read all of *Ageless Intensity*. I will eventually, but really I'm in no hurry.

That's because I read Pete McCall's 2019 book *Smarter Workouts*, and I am still using things from that book, which is why I am in no rush here. In fact, I would suggest that you not rush either. I'd even go so far as to tell you to not read this book until you have read *Smarter Workouts*. And I mean really *read* it. Make notes, put it to use, practice, push, and get uncomfortable applying the information in *Smarter Workouts*. Then, read *Ageless Intensity* and merge the material. That's what I am going to do.

You see, *Smarter Workouts* gives you a solid foundation of program design concepts to improve mobility, core strength, and metabolic conditioning. It's comprehensive, easy to use, and applicable for most people. Now I can hear Pete screaming the immortal words of Ron Popeil, "But wait, there's more!" from the top of Mount Fitness. And believe me—Pete has climbed his way to the top of that mount as he's worked with hundreds of clients.

Ageless Intensity explains how to use high-intensity exercise as we age. Wait, we're aging? Hmm . . . news to me. Regardless, it shows you how training with intensity (heavy resistance training, HIIT, explosive power training, etc.) can mitigate the effects of the aging process. Hold the phone. "Mitigate"? As in "make less severe, serious, or painful"? OK, I'm listening. So training with these principles is our fountain of youth? I'm in. Keep talking. Now, nowhere does it say it will be easy. Nowhere does it say it will be fun. But I'm OK with that. I think "easy" is a mindset, and I bring my own fun. I'm not scared. In fact, I'm fired up now. And now I'm set on digging in. I'll take what I learned in *Smarter Workouts*, add this high-intensity exercise from *Ageless Intensity*, and apply it with my clients to help them slow the aging process!

Thank you, Pete, for adding quality to the fitness landscape and for helping make trainers better. "A rising tide lifts all boats," as John F. Kennedy said in 1963. Pete McCall is that tide in fitness in 2021.

—Gunnar Peterson, CSCS

Acknowledgments

There are a number of people I would like to thank and acknowledge for helping turn *Ageless Intensity* from a vision into a reality. To Becky and Jeff and the entire team at Core Health & Fitness: Thank you for the opportunity to work with the best products and people in our industry. To Monica: Thank you for all of your support over the years; this would not have been possible without you. To all of the fitness educators, personal trainers, group fitness instructors, and strength coaches I have had the privilege of working with throughout my career: Thank you for inspiring and motivating me to learn more about the human body and how it functions. To the multitude of scientists conducting research to understand how aging changes the human body and what we can do to extend our life span: A huge thank you for your work. To listeners of the All About Fitness podcast: Thank you for your time and for providing me with the opportunity to share what I learn about how exercise can enhance the quality of life. To TMM: Thank you for your friendship and encouragement. Finally, to Michelle, Hannah, and the entire team at Human Kinetics: Thank you for your tireless efforts in keeping the ball rolling over the course of a chaotic and tumultuous year.

Introduction

To understand how I first became interested in exercise and aging, I first need to share a story about my two grandfathers.

Both of my grandfathers grew up on farms in the early 20th century; my paternal grandfather, Harold, grew up in Nebraska, while my maternal grandfather, John, was raised in New Mexico. Growing up on a farm means moving from sunup to sundown, so each man had a solid ethic of being physically active and working hard. During the Second World War, both grandfathers worked in airplane factories, and that's where their stories diverge: Grandpa John fell off a rigging and suffered a bad back injury that affected him throughout his life. After the war, he worked in the sheet metal trade and became a heating, ventilation, and air-conditioning (HVAC) mechanic, which meant a life of hauling heavy equipment and climbing on roofs despite the injury sustained in the factory. In contrast, Grandpa Harold continued working in a factory and became a floor supervisor, which meant that he was on his feet but not performing physical labor all day long; he got his physical activity from purposeful exercise outside of his workday.

Both grandfathers retired before I was born. When Grandpa Harold would come for a visit, he would do push-ups and sit-ups every morning as well as take a long walk at some point during the day. Meanwhile, Grandpa John's activity was hampered by arthritis and his back injury; he would do things with us, but he would have to push through the physical discomfort. In his later years, Grandpa John became much less active and developed type 2 diabetes, which resulted in a bilateral amputation of his legs that confined him to a wheelchair for the last years of his life. While Grandpa Harold spent his later years in a full-care facility, he was able to get out for his walk almost every day.

The difference between how my two grandfathers spent the later years of their lives is what has motivated me to learn as much as possible about exercise and the aging process. Type 2 diabetes is a disease caused, in part, by a lack of physical activity. There is no way to know with 100 percent certainty whether Grandpa John's injuries resulted in the diabetes that led to the loss of his legs, but that disease greatly affected his quality of life as he got older. Aging is going to happen; there is nothing we can do to stop the aging process, but we *do* have a choice in *how* we age. Once we are over 40, exercise becomes our means for controlling aging and reducing the effects of time on our bodies—and this book will teach you how to do just that.

Most exercise resources for the over-40 crowd focus on exercise for health, but not this one. *Ageless Intensity* will show you how high-intensity exercise can not only promote good health but also help reduce the effects of time. If you're reading this, I'm assuming that you're already exercising on a regular basis. *Ageless Intensity* is for those of you who love to exercise hard and push yourselves to your limits but want to know how to do it safely and minimize the risk of injury. If you're new to exercise or have a history of intermittent exercise—starting and stopping various programs over the years—this book can help you, but my other book, *Smarter Workouts: The Science of Exercise Made Simple*, would be a much better resource because it teaches you how to design exercise programs using only one piece of equipment. This book assumes that you like to push yourself and tend to feel a bit out of sorts if you're not a little sore the day after a hard workout (the good sore of muscles having been pushed beyond their comfort zone, that is; not the bad sore of pain revealing that something has gone wrong). What you learn here will help you to understand how high-intensity exercise influences the aging process and, most importantly, why you should challenge yourself to work out as hard as possible two or three times every week.

Nineteen ninety-eight marked the start of my full-time career in the fitness industry; however, I took my first fitness-related job in 1990 as a senior in high school. Rather than simply join a gym, I talked my way into working as a floor trainer at a now defunct Bally Total Fitness health club in suburban Maryland. Somehow my experience as a high school football player qualified me to take others through workouts. A few things about that experience stand out in my memory: (1) I was not at all qualified to be leading people through workouts; (2) there was no formal education or onboarding process for trainers before they started working on the fitness floor, which is scary considering that exercise can be fatal if done incorrectly; and (3) this is where I first observed that there was a population of die-hard exercise enthusiasts over the age of 40 who were committed to getting results from their exercise programs. (Note that I was in high school at the time, so anyone out of college seemed old to me.)

My teenage interest in gaining muscle to bulk up has led to a career of traveling the world conducting education seminars for fitness professionals while representing some of the top brands in the fitness industry. Along the way, I have continued to notice what I observed in my first fitness job back in 1990: that there is a healthy population of exercise enthusiasts who are dedicated to getting results from working out no matter how old they are.

For most adults who do not exercise, the body starts changing during the fourth decade of life (the 30s), which is when hormone levels change, cardiorespiratory efficiency declines, and the body starts losing muscle more rapidly. It's well established that exercise provides numerous benefits for promoting health by reducing the risk of chronic medical conditions like type 2 diabetes and high cholesterol. However, researchers are beginning to observe that exercise, specifically high-intensity exercise, can slow down the effects of the biological aging process, which is the degradation of physiological functions that occurs in response to the passage of time and influenced by other factors including lifestyle habits like physical activity, nutrition, or sleep. Due in part to a rapidly aging population and a cohort of active adults who have been exercising most of their lives, exercise scientists are learning that the same high-intensity exercise that can burn fat and build lean muscle mass can also change human physiology in a way that reduces the effects of time.

The current fitness boom can trace its roots back to the 1970s, when group fitness first became popular and phones were still attached to the walls in our homes. Dance aerobics became extremely popular and was promoted as a way to look great and achieve good health. The membership model for health clubs changed, making them more accessible; they transformed from hangouts for a marginalized subculture of hard-core weightlifting enthusiasts to mainstream service businesses open to everyone who could pay the membership fees. Finally, an eccentric inventor named Arthur Jones invented the Nautilus strength training machines that made exercising with resistance safe and accessible for all able-bodied adults. (Note: At the time of writing, I'm fortunate to be working as a consultant for Nautilus, Inc., and am responsible for creating the programs used to teach fitness professionals how to use their products.)

Now that we're in the third decade of the 21st century, if you're currently in your 50s, 60s, or beyond, you have grown up with the modern fitness industry. To those of you who have been exercising most of your adult lives, congratulations: You are in the first generation of active adults who have had access to gyms and exercise throughout their life span, and guess what? It shows! The original intent of exercise was to sculpt attractive bodies of lean, well-defined muscle. As the first generation of lifelong exercisers has aged, scientists have had the opportunity to study how exercise affects the aging process. What we are learning is that exercise, especially high-intensity exercise, just may be the fountain of youth that has eluded generations of explorers.

It was once thought that exercise was too strenuous for older adults or that if they did exercise, it should be at a very low intensity. That's probably because researchers did not want to risk injuring older adults in a study group by challenging them to exercise at a higher intensity. Therefore, there was no opportunity to collect data. Science has shown that exercise is good for you, but right now is the first time researchers have the opportunity to study older adults who have exercised a majority of their life span to see how it affects them and the normal biological aging process. Now, not only is there a wide body of evidence suggesting that exercise is good for older adults, but as you will read in the following pages, high-intensity exercise may yield important benefits beyond those derived from low- or moderate-intensity exercise.

When it comes to the human aging process, there are two options: (1) accept it and let nature take its course or (2) fight it. From plastic surgery to Botox injections to anti-aging clinics that specialize in prescribing hormone injections, adults around the world spend billions of dollars every year on products and services that purport to fight the effects of time on the human body. Aging is an inevitable part of the human experience that ultimately culminates in death. However, the right type of exercise program can produce numerous benefits that minimize the physiological effects of aging to allow you to maintain the energy level of adults many years younger. As you will read, high-intensity exercise could stimulate the production of anabolic hormones that promote muscle growth, and therefore can function as a literal fountain of youth. Much like death and taxes, aging is an unavoidable part of life. But as we get older, we can minimize its effects by exercising and making healthy lifestyle choices.

If, like me, you were born after 1960, you should realize that we are in the first generation of adults who have been exercising our whole lives. Yes, the baby boomers were a part of the fitness boom of the 1970s and 1980s, but if you are a member of Generation X, then there is a chance that you've been active your whole life and exercising ever since your teenage years in the 1980s when an explosion of action hero movies made big muscles popular. Think about the films of our youth such as *Rocky*. Movies like this had guys who sported muscular physiques that allowed them to kick butt and get the girl at the end. Of course, that was the motivation for the guys; 1980s pop-culture icons like Madonna and Cher, two of the first female celebrities to use personal trainers, changed the image of femininity, which resulted in the explosive growth of women starting to exercise in order to achieve the lean and fit bodies of the stars. With motivation like that, who wouldn't want to start making regular exercise a priority?

I was born in 1972, which places me right in the middle of Generation X, the population of adults born between 1965 and 1980. From technology to entertainment to design, Gen X has reshaped the world, helping to create many of the modern conveniences most of us take for granted. One major contribution of my peer group has been to reinvent physical activity and sporting competitions with the evolution of extreme sports like snowboarding, mountain biking, and skateboarding. Even though the members of Gen X are now between 40 and 60, many do not want to slow down or stop favorite physical activities that we've been enjoying since Ronald Reagan was in the White House. This book is for all of us who want to continue riding, surfing, skiing, and skateboarding no matter how old we become. In other words, consider this book a guide for how to stay in shape to enjoy your favorite activities for the rest of your life.

With the explosion of social media and video sites like YouTube and Vimeo, exercise is now more popular than ever. If you are in your 40s or beyond, it's time to shift the focus of your workouts from enhancing your appearance to developing the strength, stamina, and agility to participate in your favorite activities and live life to the fullest. The challenge is, where do you go to get good information? Can Insta-fit personalities who look great but are only in their 20s or 30s provide exercise guidance that is relevant to those of us in our 40s, 50s, or beyond? The answer is no. In my career, I have created education content for some of the top organizations in the fitness industry. If they trust me to help promote their products through evidence-based education, then you can trust that I have your best interests in mind and that all the information in this book is fully sourced and legitimate.

To help you understand how exercise affects your body—and, more importantly, how aging affects your body—this book will draw analogies to and provide insights from 1980s movies to explain the science. From *Rocky* to *The Terminator* to *Back to the Future*, popular movies can provide useful metaphors about how exercise influences the aging process.

PART I

Slow the Aging Process

1

Functional Training Redefined

Have you ever wondered how the trendy workouts that make you sweat became popular in the first place? Why is indoor cycling a thing? Who came up with the idea of high-intensity interval training (HIIT)? Did these workouts become popular because a researcher in a lab coat identified their health benefits or because a well-known celebrity extolled their virtues on a talk show? The old riddle asks, "Which came first, the chicken or the egg?" In fitness, this riddle could be rephrased: "Which came first, a popular trend or the research that validates the benefits of that trend?" There is no specific formula for how a fitness trend becomes mainstream, but if there is one common thread among popular modes of exercise, it's that they can be fun to do while producing the results people want. This chapter will help you to understand why you do the workouts that make you sweat and where the fitness industry is heading in the coming years.

The Past 25 Years in Fitness Trends

Whether you are a fitness enthusiast, a consumer of fitness services, or a fitness professional (a term that includes both personal trainers and group instructors), if you are over 40, you've witnessed an evolution of the fitness industry since the late 1990s. Over the past two decades, a number of trends have influenced how we sweat. While not a comprehensive list, here are some of the ways the industry has shifted and influenced how we exercise:

- *1970s to today*—Bodybuilding workouts that use machines and isolation exercises to develop well-defined lean muscle helped launch the modern fitness industry in the 1970s. While bodybuilding has evolved over the years, the subculture of exercise purely to enhance the human physique is a mainstay of the fitness industry that will always influence how people work out (figure 1.1).

- *Late 1990s to mid-2000s*—This was the era of functional training, in which the purpose of exercise was to improve proprioception, the ability of the central nervous system (CNS) to collect sensory information from the environment to enhance muscle activation. This chapter will cover this era in a little more depth.

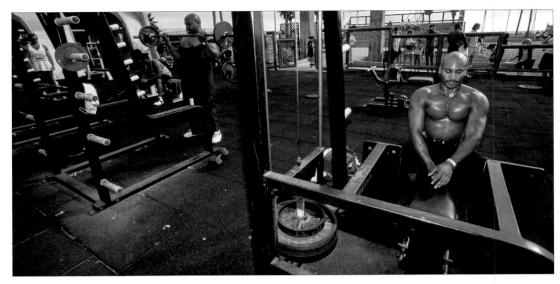

Figure 1.1 Bodybuilding will always be a popular mode of fitness, but it is not the only way to exercise.
Francis DEMANGE/Gamma-Rapho via Getty Images

- *Mid-2000s to late 2010s*—This was the era of high-intensity workout programs using a variety of equipment, including barbells, kettlebells (figure 1.2), jump boxes, and heavy medicine balls to focus on general physical preparation, the technical term for exercise to improve overall fitness without a specific, well-defined outcome. Competition-based high-intensity workout programs became so popular that the finals were broadcast on ESPN.
- *Late 2000s to 2020 (and most likely beyond)*—Obstacle course racing (OCR), a new type of running event that required participants to climb obstacles, slog through mud, and complete grueling physical challenges, rapidly gained in popularity. The popularity of OCR was due in part to the trend in high-intensity exercise. OCR created a unique experience that allowed adults young and old to test their toughness and overall fitness in events based not only on competition but also on a sense of community and shared purpose.

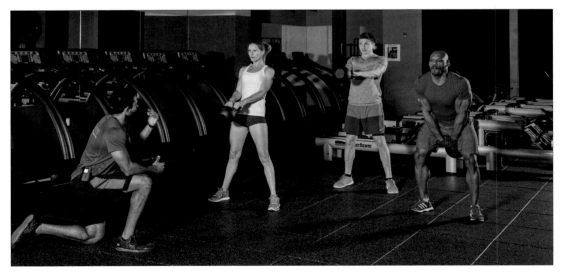

Figure 1.2 In the 2000s, high-intensity workouts with equipment like kettlebells became a popular mode of fitness because they delivered the results consumers wanted.

- *Early 2010s to 2020 (and most likely beyond)*—In this time frame, consumers shifted away from large, multipurpose health clubs to flock to boutique fitness studios that focused on a specific mode of exercise featuring workouts such as yoga, barre, indoor cycling (figure 1.3), or high-intensity circuit training.
- *Late 2010s to ????*—Social media and the introduction of online, workout-on-demand, and live-streaming services changed the way consumers gained access to top fitness instructors. Previously, an instructor had to have a company willing to spend tens of thousands of dollars to produce an exercise video, which was then sold individually to consumers. Access to high-quality video cameras on cell phones, combined with the ease of uploading content to social media platforms, changed how top fitness instructors delivered workout programs to consumers. Social media and online video platforms allow consumers to experience challenging, instructor-led workouts from the comfort of their own homes.

Yes, some of these time periods overlap; that's because some trends gain in popularity as others fall out of vogue. A number of factors influence how certain modes of exercise become more or less popular, including how media covers the fitness industry and which celebrities promote a particular type of exercise that they claim helped to change their appearance. Here's an example of how celebrities can help fuel a fitness trend: By the mid-2000s, the interest in indoor cycling had fallen off so much that a large health club company in the United States stopped building indoor cycling studios in new locations. However, in the late 2000s, popular television hostess Kelly Ripa credited indoor cycling with helping her maintain her fit physique. This led to a resurgent interest in the activity, and by the early 2010s, boutique indoor cycling studios became one of the hottest trends in fitness.

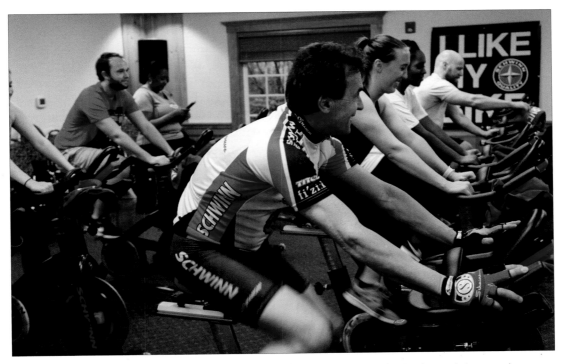

Figure 1.3 Indoor cycling is an example of a trend that looked like it was waning only to experience an explosive resurgence of popularity in the early 2010s.

The fact is that a trend becomes popular either because it produces the results consumers want or because consumers *perceive* that it works to deliver desired outcomes. Here's something to consider: Very rarely does scientific research precede a trend. More often than not, a particular mode of fitness becomes popular before exercise scientists conduct the studies to understand how it affects the human body.

However, as workout programs and modes of exercise have changed over the years, one thing has *not* changed, and that's the forward progression of time. Regardless of our relationship with the fitness industry and how long we have been exercising, we are all now a little older than when we first walked through the doors of a fitness facility. What research is starting to uncover is that not only can high-intensity exercise help burn calories and shape lean muscle, but it could also help slow down the effects of aging on our bodies. The purpose of this book is to help you understand the science of how functional training and high-intensity exercise programs may actually mitigate the effects of the biological aging process, allowing you to enjoy your favorite activities for another 25 years or hopefully much, much longer.

Training for Our Favorite Activities as We Age

Running. Hiking. Bicycling. Stand-up paddling. Swimming. Martial arts. Working out with weights and machines. These are all activities popular with adults over 40. According to the *2019 Physical Activity Council Participation Report*, approximately 60 percent of baby boomers (those born between 1945 and 1964) and 65 percent of Generation X (those born between 1965 and 1980) participate in "fitness sports," which includes exercise with weights, group fitness classes, and the use of cardio equipment. Additionally, 40 percent of baby boomers and 50 percent of Gen Xers participate in "outdoor sports" such as hiking, surfing, cycling, snowboarding, trail running, triathlons, and mountain biking (Physical Activity Council 2019). This survey shows that we're not quitting the activities we really enjoy even as we get older. Chances are that you participate in one or more of those activities and that one of the main reasons you exercise is so that you can continue enjoying them—which raises the question: "Do you want to do your favorite activity to stay in shape, or do you want to stay in shape to enjoy your favorite activity?" There is nothing wrong with participating in a specific activity like hiking or tennis if you are using that as a means to exercise; however, an exercise program that complements that activity could reduce your risk of injury and help you enjoy it on a much deeper level. Mobility exercises, strength training, and metabolic conditioning can help you develop the physical ability to be able to enjoy your favorite activities well into your later years.

Redefining Functional Training

Taking a functional approach to exercise can give you the strength and energy to achieve optimal enjoyment from your favorite activities even if exercise itself is your favorite activity; however, this requires defining the concept of functional training. The initial functional training trend in the late 1990s and early 2000s focused more on improving the balance and coordination than on the types of exercise that produce strong, powerful muscles. Personal trainers spent their time creating "functional" workout programs for their clients that focused more on complexity than on intensity. Yes, these functional workout programs could develop strong core muscles and good balance, but because of their lack of intensity, they did not produce the lean, muscular bodies that fitness consumers really wanted.

As with many trends, what began with good intent—using balance-based exercises to improve body awareness, coordination, and movement skill—ended up becoming completely overused, and by the mid-2000s, fitness consumers grew tired of balancing on air-filled half-balls. When CrossFit, a program predicated on high-intensity exercise, was introduced in the mid-2000s, it instantly exploded in popularity because fitness enthusiasts quickly realized that intensity, heavy weights, explosive power training, and conditioning to the point of fatigue were necessary for achieving the lean, muscular physiques they desired.

As high-intensity workouts became the norm, fitness consumers began incorporating explosive exercises, including barbell lifts such as the snatch and the clean and jerk, kettlebell swings, heavy medicine ball throws, and box jumps, into their workout programs. Once almost exclusively the domain of elite athletes training for competition, these exercises require rapid muscle force production, which in turn creates the stimulus for muscle growth. A little side note: Up until the mid-2000s, Olympic weightlifting platforms (figure 1.4) were almost nonexistent at commercial health clubs and could be found primarily in performance training facilities or in the weight rooms used for collegiate athletic programs. High-intensity barbell training has now become so popular with general fitness consumers that it is difficult to find a modern health club or fitness facility that doesn't have at least one platform in the weightlifting area.

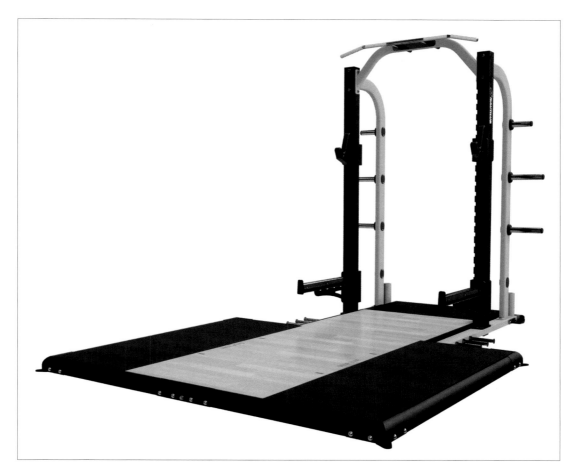

Figure 1.4 Olympic weightlifting platform.

To paraphrase the *Oxford English Dictionary*'s definition of *functional*, it refers to an object having a specific activity, purpose, or task. A different way to look at that would be an object designed for the purpose of being practical and useful as opposed to attractive. In the early 2000s, functional training took this definition literally, with workouts that emphasized coordination over force production. The goal of many of these "functional" workouts was to develop improved body awareness instead of muscle definition or overall strength. From aerial yoga to Zumba classes, the problem with any workout program that focuses too much on only one kind of exercise is it leads to repetitive stress that can cause an injury. Either that, or your body adapts to the stimulus and stops responding. The early 2000s version of functional training helped consumers move better but failed to produce the well-defined muscles and lean bodies they wanted. High-intensity workouts, while effective for muscle growth and fat burning, have a different problem: Do them too often, and there is a high likelihood that you will either become injured from doing the same movements too often or get stuck on a plateau because your body stops responding.

Truly Functional Training

Functional training has reemerged in the fitness lexicon, but it now refers to programs that include exercises for mobility, strength, power, and metabolic conditioning, along with consideration for the recovery period after the workout when muscles adapt to the demands imposed during exercise and become stronger. Taking the definition a step further, functional training could also refer to how exercise programs can be designed using these components to slow down the effects of the normal biological aging process. Ever since fitness became popular back in the 1970s, the most common reasons people started exercising were to get rid of unwanted weight, increase strength, add muscle size, or improve muscle definition. These can all be achieved with the components of functional training—namely, exercises for mobility, strength, power, and metabolic conditioning. Your challenge is learning how to design and execute workouts that produce these results in the fastest, safest, most effective ways possible.

For example, strength training with heavy resistance develops and maintains the muscle mass that many consumers want. However, if done too often or incorrectly, it can cause an injury. One significant factor in the redefinition of functional training is an aging population of consumers who want to continue their favorite activities but need to learn that mobility training and recovery strategies influence their results as much as, if not more than, the workouts themselves. Learning how to balance high-intensity exercise with mobility training and effective recovery strategies could help you to get the results you want while avoiding unnecessary injuries. It is necessary to enhance movement skill to remain injury-free both in and out of the gym environment, yet this is an often-overlooked component of many fitness programs. The most effective fitness professionals and exercise programs teach proper movement skill and exercise technique first before progressing to the high-intensity exercise responsible for adding muscle and burning fat. Educated fitness professionals know that moving well and maintaining proper mobility are the foundation for achieving long-term results from high-intensity exercise. As Dr. Kelly Starrett, a physical therapist, a CrossFit coach, and the author of the book *Becoming a Supple Leopard* wrote, "Mobility is the first step in moving better. If you understand how to move correctly, you can mitigate movement errors that have the potential to cause injury" (Starrett 2015).

This new approach to functional training comes with a solid understanding that exercise by itself is not enough to achieve results. In addition to the workouts, functional training programs should feature postexercise recovery strategies, which can include mobility exercises, myofascial release with equipment such as foam rollers or rolling sticks to reduce muscle tightness, heat exposure in a sauna, cold exposure in a cryotherapy chamber, and the most effective recovery strategy of all, high-quality sleep. *Functional* is defined as being task specific. For aging fitness fanatics who want to continue exercising well into their later years, the primary task of a functional training exercise program is a proper application of intensity, mobility training, and recovery in a way that slows the effects of the aging process. In this context, *functional training* can be defined as the use of high-intensity exercise combined with mobility training and recovery strategies to slow the effects of the biological aging process.

If I Can Change, You Can Change

The 1985 movie *Rocky IV* provides an excellent example of functional training. It was released at the height of the Cold War between the United States and the former Soviet Union. In the movie, Rocky seeks to avenge his friend's death by agreeing to fight Soviet boxer Ivan Drago in Drago's home country. To prepare for the fight, Rocky travels to the Soviet Union and trains in a barn in what looks to be the frozen tundra of Siberia, while Drago, the robotic product of Soviet sport scientists, exercises in a state-of-the-art facility surrounded by the latest technology.

The film includes a staple feature of 1980s movies: a montage set to a fast-paced soundtrack, this one depicting Rocky doing pull-ups and inverted sit-ups on a rafter in a barn, lifting and pushing a cart, carrying logs, and running through snow. These scenes of Rocky training for his fight are a perfect example of functional training because they show a variety of different exercises to develop the strength, power, endurance, and agility our hero will need to defeat his Soviet adversary. Of course, Rocky, representing the United States, defeats Drago, the symbol of the former Soviet Union. During the course of the fight, the crowd stops cheering for Drago to root for the "Italian Stallion" (Rocky's nickname). The movie ends with Rocky making a stirring speech about world peace by referencing how the crowd changed from cheering for the Soviet fighter to cheering for him. "If I can change, and you can change, everybody can change," is what Rocky bellowed into the microphone as he was declared the victor. It was an inspiring statement about peace between the two adversaries and one of the most memorable scenes of the movie. Besides being an uplifting statement about world peace, little did the producers of the movie know that they had created the perfect juxtaposition between functional training and the machine-based exercise programs that can produce a muscular, lean body that looks good but may not be able to function effectively at the highest levels of human performance.

Here's another great example to help you understand this new approach to functional training. In the 1986 film *Highlander*, Christopher Lambert stars as Connor MacLeod, an immortal who does not experience the effects of time on his body. The theme of the movie is that a contingent of immortals is engaged in a contest throughout time, battling each other to the death until only one remains. Throughout the centuries, these immortals challenge each other in sword fights, and the only way they can be eliminated is to have his or her head chopped off. Like the training

Rocky did for his fight, sword fighting is an example of high-intensity exercise that, in the case of Connor MacLeod, can literally have an age-defying effect on the body.

To be successful as a warrior, MacLeod needs an extreme amount of functional training, specifically the strength to control a heavy sword, the mobility to dodge an attacker, the conditioning to sustain a lengthy fight, the explosive power to swing a sword with enough force to remove an opponent's head, and the ability to recover quickly in order to be prepared to vanquish the next foe. Maybe one reason why Connor MacLeod was able to maintain his youth through the ages was the high-intensity exercise he did while engaged in combat against the other immortals. While you're not in a battle with opponents to the death, think about the aging process as a battle to retain the physical abilities you need in order to enjoy your favorite activities. If you train for the same strength, mobility, stamina, and power it takes to be victorious in a sword fight, you can achieve victory in your fight against the effects that time can have on your body.

A truly functional training workout program includes all of the following modalities of exercise, most of which can be seen in these classic 1980s movies: the strength to lift heavy weights, the mobility to move the body through multiple movement patterns, the metabolic conditioning to increase endurance and delay the onset of fatigue, and the power to perform explosive actions. The one component overlooked by these movies was the postexercise recovery that can help the body heal and prepare for the demands of the workout. The good news is that it is completely possible to exercise using the same methods demonstrated by Rocky and Connor MacLeod without having to step in a ring or risk having your head removed by another immortal.

An Accumulating Body of Evidence

Prior to the mid-2000s, very few people participated in high-intensity exercise with any regularity. For the most part, high-intensity workouts were performed by well-conditioned athletes preparing for the rigors of their competition. Most of the research conducted on high-intensity exercise had been done almost exclusively in the context of how to help athletes condition more effectively for a particular sport. For example, one of the most popular methods of HIIT is the Tabata protocol, which calls for 20 seconds of extremely high-intensity exercise followed by 10 seconds of passive recovery repeated for eight cycles over a four-minute period. Tabata intervals have become a staple of HIIT programs, yet the original purpose of the research Dr. Izumi Tabata conducted in the mid-1990s was to see whether short bouts of high-intensity exercise would allow members of the Japanese speedskating team to improve their aerobic capacity without having to perform a high volume of conditioning (Tabata et al. 1997).

Remember that research is often conducted *after* a fitness trend becomes popular? As high-intensity exercise became popular with the average fitness consumer in the mid- to late 2000s (figure 1.5), exercise scientists began to study its effects on the general population. As high-intensity exercise for health benefits has received further study, more and more findings have been published, and the evidence is accumulating that the same kinds of high-intensity exercise that can help an athlete like Rocky prepare for competition at the highest levels of a sport can also provide important health benefits for most people, including mitigating many of the effects of the biological aging process (Katula, Rejeski, and Marsh 2008; Volaklis, Halle, and Meisinger 2015; Fragala et al. 2019).

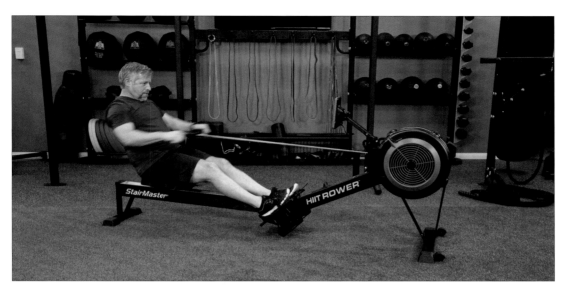

Figure 1.5 High-intensity workouts can be performed using a variety of equipment, including rowing machines.

In other words, don't let aging happen to you. Train like an athlete, and while you may not become an immortal like Connor MacLeod, the evidence suggests that high-intensity exercise can indeed slow down the effects of time on your body. Instead of using exercise as something to make you look better, recognize exercise for what it truly is: an activity that can help you add years of high-quality living so that you can experience maximal enjoyment out of the later years of your life. The good news is that many of the high-intensity barbell, kettlebell, and metabolic conditioning workouts that can help change your body are also functional for the task of slowing the effects of time.

Five Components of Functional Training

A truly functional training exercise program should organize your workouts in a way that allows you to maintain your overall level of conditioning as you age and should include the following training components:

- *Mobility. Flexibility* refers to the range of motion (ROM) allowed by a joint. *Extensibility* refers to the ability of muscle and elastic connective tissue to lengthen and shorten. Motor control is how the CNS organizes your muscular actions to control movement. Mobility is a combination of optimal joint ROM, tissue extensibility, and motor control—more specifically, the ability to organize and coordinate the body's movements through space.

- *Strength. Force* is defined as the product of a mass and its acceleration. When a muscle contracts, it accelerates a mass, resulting in a force; strength comes from the ability of muscle fibers to generate force while contracting against an external resistance. The CNS communicates with a muscle via the motor unit, which is a motor neuron and the muscle fibers connected to it. When the motor neuron is activated, it signals the attached muscle fibers to contract, which generates the force for movement. Strength training can increase the number of motor units activated in a muscle (Zatsiorsky, Kraemer, and Fry 2021).

- *Power.* The product of force and velocity, power is the velocity of force production. While strength and power are related, they are actually separate traits that need to be developed independently. Strength is the amount of force produced, while power is the velocity of muscle force production. More specifically, it's the speed at which muscle motor units innervate their attached muscle fibers to cause a contraction. Due to atrophy of type II (fast-twitch) muscle fibers, the loss of muscle power could have a greater impact on quality of life than the loss of strength (Bet da Rosa Orssatto et al. 2019).

- *Metabolic conditioning.* Commonly referred to as cardiorespiratory exercise, metabolic conditioning increases the efficiency of the body's metabolic system, which processes the carbohydrates and fats from food into the chemical form of energy that fuels muscle contractions. HIIT is a time-efficient mode of metabolic conditioning that not only can help burn calories but may also help produce the anabolic hormones responsible for growing lean muscle, an important component in reducing the effects of time on the body. While HIIT can produce results, too much of it without proper recovery can lead to overtraining. For this reason, it is important to include other types of metabolic conditioning. Steady-state training (SST) features a high volume of work to enhance aerobic capacity. Low-intensity interval training (LIIT) uses low- to moderate-intensity intervals combined with periods of active rest to improve the efficiency of the cardiorespiratory system to deliver oxygen to working muscles. Variable (duration) interval training (VIT) alternates between short, intermediate, and long periods of work to challenge the body to work efficiently for different lengths of time. In addition, variable-intensity interval training (VIIT) alternates between periods of low-, moderate-, and high-intensity exercise to provide an overload. Not all metabolic conditioning training has to be high intensity; using a combination of HIIT, SST, LIIT, VIT, and VIIT to vary work intervals between different levels of intensity and time durations can help ensure that you are not using any one energy system more than another when you exercise.

- *Recovery.* Recovery is the way in which tissues and other structures in the body adapt to the stresses imposed during exercise. It includes repair of damaged tissues, replacing spent energy, and allowing the nervous system to rest before being stimulated to act again.

How to Get Results From Your Workout Program

Whether you're starting a program from scratch or looking to add new ideas to your existing workouts, be careful that you don't go overboard with any one mode of exercise. A well-rounded program should include high-, moderate-, and low-intensity exercises so that your body never adapts to any particular level of intensity. To produce results, an exercise program does not need to be overly complicated, with different exercises for each body part. It does, however, need to provide an adequate stimulus to initiate physiological changes in the body. Free weights. Machines. Kettlebells. Heavy medicine balls. Bodyweight. There is not one single piece of equipment that is most effective for the high-intensity exercise necessary to slow aging. For best results, an exercise program for functional training as defined in this chapter should seek to use all types of equipment but at different times and for different reasons. For example, bodyweight training can be extremely effective for improving mobility, while kettlebells can help develop explosive power or burn calories through metabolic conditioning, and machines can help enhance strength by isolating one muscle group at a time.

Doing the same exercises repeatedly and always exercising at a high intensity without allowing for proper rest between workouts are examples of how exercise can be done incorrectly. As Gray Cook, a physical therapist and the author of the book *Movement*, has observed, "Current exercise programming has two inherent problems: some movements are performed too frequently or with too much intensity and movements are performed too infrequently or with too little intensity" (Cook 2010). Common injuries like tendinitis or impingement syndrome that restrict joint motion could result from doing the same exercises too often. Overtraining is an accumulation of physical stress because the body does not have the opportunity to fully recover after exercise. Truly functional training addresses not only the exercises performed in the workout but also the postexercise recovery strategies that are important for remaining injury-free. Recovery strategies allow the body to adapt to the imposed stresses of exercise, helping to promote the desired adaptations to improve overall health and functional strength.

Yes, you will receive numerous health benefits if you exercise regularly at a low or moderate intensity; but unless you incorporate high-intensity strength training, power training, and metabolic conditioning into your workouts along with specific postexercise strategies, you may not experience the greatest benefits your fitness efforts could deliver. The following chapters will address the research that suggests that high-intensity, heavy-resistance training and power training not only are safe for us as we age, but are a recommended method for greatly improving strength and efficiency in many activities of daily living (ADLs), and that high-intensity exercise should be an integral component of workout programs well into our later years.

2

Change How You Age

"Aging is a degenerative process affecting virtually all known organisms that is characterized by progressive deterioration of cellular components and deregulation of cellular processes, resulting in mortality" (Masoro and Austad 2011). Okay, that's a glum assessment, but the one certainty in life is that it will eventually culminate in death. Aging has been studied as a specific science, known as gerontology, only since the 1940s, which means that there is about a 30-year gap between the beginning of the study of how aging affects the body and the start of the modern fitness industry. For most older adults, aging results in less time participating in physical activities like exercise and more time in sedentary positions. For this reason, most of the research on aging has been conducted primarily on older adults who do not participate in much, if any, physical activity. Now having access to older adults who have been physically active their entire lives, researchers are starting to compile data on how years of regular, consistent exercise affect human biology during the aging process.

There are a number of different theories about what causes aging, a natural process that affects most of the systems in the body. This chapter will focus on the effects of the aging process on the systems in our body related to exercise and on what science is starting to learn about how exercise, specifically high-intensity exercise, can mitigate or even reverse these effects. There appear to be two key factors that we can change that could allow us to add years to our life span: the environment and exercise (McDonald 2019).

Where you live can have an important impact on the aging process. Factors include weather, which may promote outdoor physical activity; traffic; pollution; available jobs; access to health care; and quality of food sources. As humans we have varying abilities to select an optimal environment that can reduce stressors and allow us to thrive. However, since this is a book on exercise, we will focus on how exercise can influence the aging process, specifically how we age and whether we can design exercise programs that allow us to increase our life expectancy.

Life Span and Life Expectancy

Life span is the length of time from when we are born to when we die, and the good news is that there is an accumulating body of evidence suggesting that exercise in general, and high-intensity exercise in particular, can add years of high-quality living to our life span. Life expectancy is the average length of time that a human is expected to live and is based on the experiences of others the same general age and demographic (Taylor and Johnson 2008). From the 16th to late 19th century, the average life span for adults in the United States hovered between 35 and 45. In the 20th century, we started understanding a lot more about how to promote health and fight various diseases that could cause early death. As a result, in the early years of the 21st century the average life expectancy for American adults was 80 years for females and 76 for males (McDonald 2019). We can now live much longer than any other humans in history—but what good are the extra years if we don't have the strength or aerobic capacity to participate in and enjoy our favorite activities?

Researchers have identified six phases of the adult life span (Taylor and Johnson 2008):

Phase	Ages (yr)
Early adulthood	20-29
Middle adulthood	30-44
Late adulthood	45-64
Elderly	65-74
Older elderly	75-84
Very old	85 and above

Tosato and colleagues (2007) identified three curves of aging: (1) disease and disability; (2) usual aging; and (3) successful aging, which is represented by minimal aging-related loss of physiological functions. When we were in early adulthood, we started to exercise for a number of reasons, such as training for sports, socializing, maintaining good health, and, of course, enhancing our appearance in an effort to be more attractive to potential mates. However, as we make the transition into late adulthood and beyond, it is essential to make an important shift in our view of exercise, specifically by coming to see that it is the means by which we can experience successful aging. Yes, an attractive appearance is always important, but once we hit our 40s and beyond the primary focus of exercise should be for controlling the aging process.

Aging will change our bodies in some ways that are inevitable. Even weightlifters who consistently use high-intensity strength training to prepare for masters-level competitions can expect to lose 1 to 1.5 percent of strength per year, with even greater losses after age 70 (Haff and Triplett 2016). Although there is nothing we can do to completely stop the aging process, the evidence suggests that high-intensity exercise can provide numerous benefits that can allow us to enjoy our favorite physical activities, including exercise itself, well into our later years.

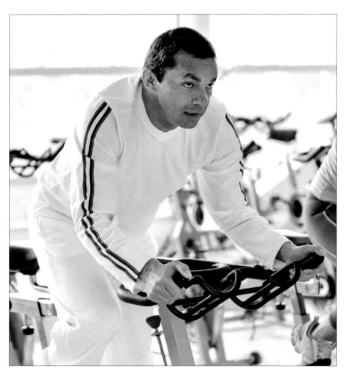

The current population of older adults who have been exercising throughout their lives is providing important insights into how exercise can slow the effects of the aging process.
Andres Rodriguez/fotolia.com

How We Age

"Although...every physiological system shows some decline with age, the amount of decline, the systems affected and the age at which the decline begins are highly variable and specific to each individual" (McDonald 2019). Just as no two snowflakes are alike, no two adults will age exactly the same way. Likewise, exercise will affect each person differently. Research can provide a general idea of the results from a particular mode of exercise, but exercise is only one variable that influences how the body changes; other factors include nutrition, sleep, and overall level of stress. Although there is no way to guarantee specific results from any exercise program, the evidence does suggest that a lack of regular physical activity is bad for your health. A sedentary lifestyle with a lack of physical activity is a risk factor for developing heart disease; in fact, the World Health Organization (WHO) estimates that globally up to 5 million deaths a year could be avoided simply by increasing levels of physical activity. In addition, the WHO suggests that individuals who do not meet the recommended levels of physical activity have a 20 to 30 percent greater risk of an early death when compared to those who perform sufficient levels of physical activity (World Health Organization). So, while there is no guarantee about the results, the evidence suggests that *not* exercising could take years off your life.

There are different ways to classify the physiological changes that occur during the aging process (table 2.1): Chronological aging cannot be controlled, but the other classifications can be altered through lifestyle choices and specific interventions like exercise (Pocari, Bryant, and Comana 2015).

From plastic surgery to Botox injections to clinics that specialize in prescribing injections of growth hormone (GH), maturing adults take extraordinary, and often painful, measures in the effort to mitigate the effects of the aging process. Chronological aging is simply the passage of time; the only way it changes is with death. However, lifestyle choices like exercise can change how the aging process affects you, allowing you to significantly increase the chances of adding years of high-quality living to your life span. You don't need to pay for expensive, painful medical procedures or uncomfortable injections of anabolic steroids; high-intensity exercise itself can minimize the effects of aging. Okay, admittedly exercising at an

Table 2.1 **Classifications of Aging**

Classification	Description
Chronological aging	The effect of aging as a function of the passage of time; it happens independent of other variables.
Biological aging	Gradual deterioration of cells, tissues, and organs within the body as the result of the passage of time; influenced by environment and lifestyle habits.
Primary aging	The progressive maturation and eventual deterioration of all physiological structures and systems, from individual cells to connective tissues to vital organs; a function of natural biology that cannot be altered.
Secondary aging	How lifestyle choices and behaviors influence the aging process; many of these factors—such as nutrition, alcohol intake, sleep, overall stress levels, and drug use—are controllable and could influence the risk of developing a disease such as type 2 diabetes, obesity, or cancer.
Active aging	An approach to aging that includes the seven dimensions of wellness (physical, intellectual, emotional, spiritual, environmental, vocational, and social) to promote overall health and wellness throughout the course of the aging process; encourages active involvement in life despite health status, disease condition, or socioeconomic status.

extremely high intensity can be uncomfortable, but that's only for a few seconds at a time, which is preferable to days of discomfort from a surgical procedure. While it is challenging, high-intensity exercise can foster active aging and mitigate the effects of both primary and secondary aging by expending unnecessary energy (body fat), promoting the growth of new cells to repair muscle and connective tissue, and stimulating the production of hormones responsible for growing muscle and burning fat. High-intensity exercise could be providing greater benefits than moderate-intensity exercise related to mitigating the aging process (Taylor 2013; Fragala et al. 2019; Rice and Keogh 2009). Which would you rather do: spend thousands of dollars a year on uncomfortable, potentially dangerous medical procedures or suffer through a couple of 30-minute high-intensity interval training (HIIT) workouts every week at your favorite fitness facility? When you add in the social benefits from friendships you could develop through the HIIT workouts, it becomes a very easy decision indeed.

What Do American Muscle Cars and Aging Have in Common?

The Dukes of Hazzard was not a movie until 2005, but it *was* a television series that ran from 1979 to 1985 on the CBS network. It provides a fitting analogy for how exercise can help us to maintain our bodies. One of the main stars of the show was a car, specifically a modified, bright orange 1969 Dodge Charger. The show took place a number of years after the car was manufactured, but the Duke boys consistently maintained the car and kept it operating at a high level of performance so that they could outrun their foes.

It's not just the souped-up Dodge Charger driven by the Duke boys—*all* muscle cars from the 1960s can provide a good analogy for how exercise slows down the effects of the aging process. From the Charger to Ford's Mustang to Chevrolet's Corvette, in the 1960s all of the major American automobile companies built cars

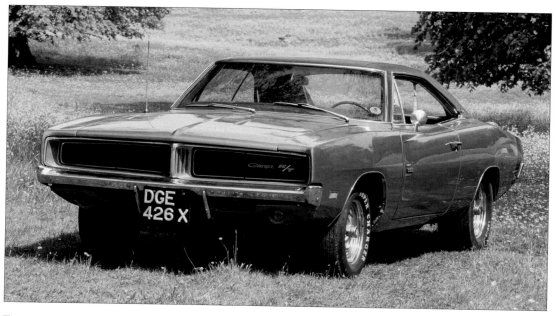

The mechanical care required to properly maintain an American muscle car from the 1960s provides a fitting analogy for how exercise can manage the effects of aging on the human body.
National Motor Museum/Heritage Images/Getty Images

that not only looked great but could really perform on the street. These muscle cars are now more than 50 years old, and those that have had regular maintenance are still functioning and capable of being driven at a high level of performance. Just as regular maintenance extends the useful life of a car, exercise improves the function of many of the physiological systems responsible for optimal health. The care required to ensure that a 50-year-old car can drive just as well now as when it first rolled off the factory floor is a fitting analogy for how exercise can maintain optimal health and reduce the effects of the aging process.

A car is designed to be driven. The engine and systems that control it are most effective when operated on a regular basis. If a car sits idle for too long, the vital fluids such as engine oil or brake fluid can settle, break down, and be unable to do their job effectively the next time the car is driven. If a car is left outside without proper protection, its paint may oxidize, tires deteriorate, and parts start to rust. On the other hand, if a car is driven and stored properly and, most importantly, maintained, then it can provide many years of safe operation and enjoyment for its owner. Exercise is your tool to keep all of the systems of your body operating at a high level.

To take the car analogy a step further, you can take great care of a car, but unless it's driven on a regular basis, the engine may not function properly when it is finally taken out on the road. Many people become less physically active as they age; if they exercise at all, it's low-intensity, "safe" activities such as walking or water aerobics. This is like keeping a car in a garage and not driving it.

Because many older adults now in their 70s first started exercising when fitness became a trend in the 1970s, researchers can now study the effects of years of exercise to see how it has changed the human aging process. In one study, researchers performed a series of tests on adults in their 70s (Gries et al. 2018). The study included three groups of older adults—one group that had participated in casual but consistent exercise throughout their life span, approximately 50 years of adulthood; one group that had regularly trained for competitive running events since the 1970s; and one group that was not very physically active. In addition, the study included a group of younger adults in their 20s so that researchers could compare tissue samples between the older adults and the younger cohort.

Study authors observed that both groups of active older adults had greater capillary density when compared to the sedentary adults of the same age. Capillaries are where the cardiorespiratory system delivers oxygen and nutrients from the blood into muscle tissue. An increase in capillaries results in more efficient oxygen exchange into muscle tissue, along

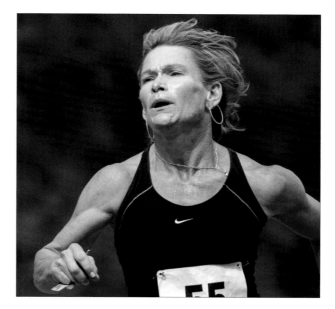

High-intensity exercise can produce a number of benefits for masters athletes that help muscles function at a high level of performance, even in the later years of the adult lifespan.

with the enzymes required to metabolize substrates into energy. Enzymes assist in converting the nutrition substrates of fat and carbohydrate into energy to fuel muscular activity. Researchers found that the active older adults had tissue samples similar to those of the younger adults and noted, "Fifty years of lifelong exercise fully preserved skeletal muscle capillarization and aerobic enzymes." This suggests that exercise helped muscle tissue to function efficiently, specifically in regard to oxygen consumption and substrate metabolism as well as the ability to communicate with other tissues (Gries et al. 2018). Both groups of active older adults exercised, on average, a minimum of four days a week, which provides powerful evidence that maintaining a high level of fitness can help muscle tissue function as if it were years younger. If you are still concerned about using exercise to help you look better, note that increasing a muscle's ability to consume oxygen via greater capillary density could allow it to retain a more pleasing appearance well into the later years, too.

The physiological systems of the human body are similar to the workings of a car in that with the proper fuel (nutrition), maintenance, and operation, a person can have a long, healthy, vibrant life full of enjoyable physical activity. In both humans and cars, the efficiency of oxygen use affects performance and extends functional life. In a muscle car like the Duke boys' Charger, you can rebuild the carburetor to enhance its performance and lengthen its life. Likewise, you can change your aerobic capacity—the maximum volume of oxygen consumed per kilogram of bodyweight, expressed as mL/kg—to literally add years of life. Gries and colleagues (2018) observed that study participants who performed higher-intensity exercise throughout their life span possessed a higher aerobic capacity than other study participants of the same age. This is an important observation because aerobic capacity quantifies oxygen consumption, which can be measured in metabolic equivalents (METs). One MET is the amount of oxygen consumed while the body is at rest, which is approximately 3.5 mL/kg. The study established that increasing aerobic capacity by one MET could result in a 13 to 15 percent reduction in the risk of all-cause mortality, which equated to a 30 percent reduction in the risk of early mortality for the active older adult groups when compared to the sedentary group (Gries et al. 2018). High-intensity exercise could help increase your aerobic capacity, allowing your cardiorespiratory system to function as it did when you were young while possibly reducing your risk of an early death.

An adult who is sedentary, makes poor nutritional choices, and participates in risky lifestyle habits such as smoking cigarettes or drinking too much alcohol could accelerate the effects of secondary aging and possibly cause a premature death, which is exactly like abandoning a car in a vacant lot. A car engine can fall into disrepair if not driven regularly, just as human muscle tissue will atrophy, become smaller, and lose the ability to generate significant amounts of force if not engaged in exercise. Sedentary adults can expect to lose 8 to 10 percent of muscle tissue per decade after they reach 40. But if you are physically active and exercise past 40, you may only experience a loss of 2 percent per decade (McDonald 2019).

The unfortunate thing is that as we get older, our cells age right along with us, and that appears to be what creates most of the changes we experience. Scientists have not been able to identify one specific mechanism that causes aging-related muscle loss; however, the evidence appears to suggest that a reduction in the efficiency of how mitochondria in muscle cells function, a decrease in the number of satellite cells used to repair damaged tissues, and an accumulation of free radicals like reactive oxygen species (ROS) and damaged proteins all play a role (Masoro and Austad 2011; McDonald 2019). Again, the car analogy can be applied; with the right amount of restoration and mechanical work, an abandoned car can be resurrected and brought back to good working order. The good news is that just as restoration can return a car to life, adjusting the intensity and volume of exercise can help maintain muscle mass and improve the ability of many of your physiological systems to function, allowing you to retain muscle tissue while improving its performance. Exercise can help control the primary aging process, but to have the greatest effects, exercise programs must alternate between periods of high, low, and moderate intensity to challenge the physiological systems to function at a high level while allowing the proper time for rest so the tissues have a chance to recover, repair, and become more efficient (figure 2.1).

Table 2.2 shows how the primary aging process affects a number of the physiological systems related to exercise and physical activity.

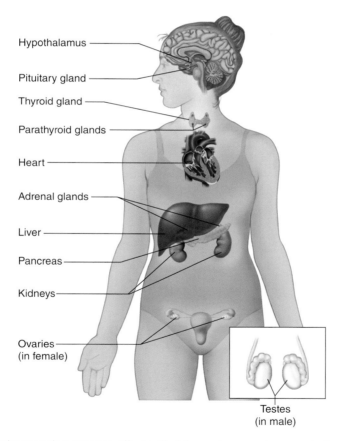

Figure 2.1 The primary aging process affects all of the systems and organs in the human body.

Table 2.2 **How the Primary Aging Process Affects Human Physiology**

Physiological system	Function	Effect of aging
Cardiorespiratory	The transportation system brings oxygen in from the air, places it in the bloodstream, and delivers it to tissues and organs; it also removes metabolic by-products and other waste (e.g., carbon dioxide), which is excreted from the body.	• The heart functions as a pump to move blood through the body; if not used regularly, it can become weaker and lose efficiency, causing a number of chronic health conditions. • Cardiac output is the product of heart rate (HR), number of beats per minute (bpm), and stroke volume (the volume of blood pumped by the left ventricle per contraction). Cardiac output can decline at a rate of 10% per decade over the age of 25. • Arteriosclerosis causes thickening of the arteries, making it more difficult for the heart to pump blood through the system. • Reduction in the number of alveoli (tiny sacs in the lungs where oxygen is withdrawn from the air and placed in the blood), capillaries (the blood vessels where oxygen is transferred to muscle tissue), and cellular mitochondria (the organelles that convert oxygen and substrates into energy for muscle activity) can reduce aerobic efficiency. • A reduced sensitivity to epinephrine and norepinephrine, the neurotransmitters responsible for energy production, is related to a 30-50% reduction in maximum heart rate between the ages of 25 and 85.
Neural/central nervous system (CNS)	The CNS has three components: sensory, integration, and motor; it determines what functions the body needs and sends the signals to initiate and control those functions.	• A low level of physical activity can cause atrophy of the type II muscle fibers responsible for strength and power. • Demyelination of nerves can result in thinning of motor neurons and reduced conductivity, leading to a loss of force production from attached muscle fibers. • Reaction time increases, slowing reflexive response to rapid changes of direction or force production. • A sedentary lifestyle can reduce the ability of the sensory system to sense what is happening in the environment to determine the appropriate motor response. • Reduced efficiency of sensory nerves could result in loss of balance, of the ability to maintain the center of mass over the base of support, and of motor control (the ability to activate the muscles necessary for coordinated movement).
Muscular	The contractile element of muscle is comprised of actin and myosin protein filaments, which generate a force when stimulated to contract by a motor neuron; the muscular system includes both type I (aerobic) and type II (anaerobic) muscle fibers.	• In sarcopenia (the loss of muscle mass), as much as 10% of muscle mass is lost per decade over the age of 30. • Because of lost muscle mass and nerve conductivity, explosive strength and power can greatly decrease over the age of 40. • Functional strength to perform necessary ADLs is reduced.
Skeletal and connective tissue	The skeletal system provides a framework for the body. The osseous structures of the skeleton and the connective tissues are composed of collagen that models along the lines of stress; connective tissue includes elastic (fascia and tendons) and inelastic (ligaments) tissues.	• Osteoporosis, the loss of bone mineral density (BMD), can affect both women *and* men, causing bones to weaken; this makes them susceptible to fracturing or breaking in an accidental fall. • As connective tissue ages, it can lose the ability to retain the water that allows different layers to successfully glide over one another during movement, making it easier for adhesions to form. • Lack of movement from a sedentary lifestyle or repetitive motions from the same exercises can increase the collagen content of muscle and connective tissues, which when combined with less hydration can result in adhesions that limit tissue extensibility and joint range of motion (ROM). • Arthritis increases inflammation of joints, which can reduce their ability to move unrestricted through the full ROM.

Physiological system	Function	Effect of aging
Metabolic	The body's metabolism digests substrates (fat, carbohydrate, and protein) and converts them into other chemicals to help fuel activity and repair damaged tissues.	• A loss of muscle mass in general and atrophy of type II muscle fibers specifically could reduce the body's ability to metabolize glucose, increasing insulin sensitivity. • A reduction of type II muscle fibers can result in lower levels of the enzymes required for anaerobic energy production. • A sedentary lifestyle could result in a loss of mitochondria in type I muscle fibers, reducing their ability to convert oxygen and free fatty acids (FFAs) into energy.
Endocrine	The endocrine system produces the hormones that regulate and control a number of cellular functions, including energy production and tissue repair.	• Andropause affects men over 35, who can experience a 1-3% loss of testosterone (T) production per year. • Menopause affects women in their 40s and beyond who experience changes that result in the loss of the menstrual cycle. • Low levels of strenuous physical activity and the loss of muscle mass can reduce the levels of anabolic hormones, specifically GH, T, and insulin-like growth factor-1, responsible for promoting tissue repair and muscle growth.
Cognitive	The cognitive system is the ability of the brain to process thoughts, synthesize information, and retain memories.	• There is a direct link between sedentary lifestyles and the onset of memory loss and diseases like Alzheimer's and dementia that reduce cognitive function. • Reduced oxygen and blood flow to brain structures could be a cause of impaired cognitive function during aging.
Emotional/social	Emotional well-being and a positive social environment are important for successful aging.	• There is a direct connection between the social isolation that can occur during aging and isolation, depression, and other mental health issues. • Belonging to a fitness facility or finding a workout partner can help establish and develop relationships with like-minded individuals of all ages, which is one factor for maintaining good health through the aging process.

Diseases Related to the Aging Process

Aging is a normal biological process, not a disease. A disease impairs optimal function of tissues, organs, or physiological systems. Starting at middle adulthood, or about 30, as physiological systems deteriorate and weaken due to the normal aging process, the risk of developing a disease or chronic health condition increases significantly. Risk factors for developing a chronic disease include a sedentary lifestyle, excess bodyweight, high amounts of stress, and excessive alcohol intake. Just as leaving a car exposed to the elements without proper long-term care will cause it to rust and fall apart, a sedentary lifestyle with minimal physical activity increases the risk of a number of chronic health conditions. Table 2.3 identifies aging-related, chronic health conditions; there is no way to develop 100 percent immunity from these conditions, but healthy habits including high-intensity exercise can significantly reduce your risk for developing one.

Table 2.3 **Chronic Health Conditions Influenced by Aging**

Disease or chronic condition	How it changes the body
Obesity	Excessive amounts of body fat can restrict joint motion, place extra stress on the heart, and lead to other conditions, such as type 2 diabetes, high blood pressure (hypertension), and cardiovascular disease.
Type 2 diabetes	Excessive weight gain and overeating can cause the metabolism to become resistant to insulin, losing the ability to properly metabolize carbohydrates into energy.
Cardiovascular disease	Impaired cardiac function can result in conditions such as hypertension and arteriosclerosis, which limit the ability of the heart to circulate blood throughout the body.
High cholesterol	An accumulation of low-density lipoprotein (LDL) cholesterol can result in arterial blockages that reduce cardiac efficiency and aerobic capacity.
Musculoskeletal diseases	Conditions such as osteoporosis (loss of BMD making bones weaker and more susceptible to breakage), sarcopenia (loss of lean muscle mass), and arthritis (inflammation of joint capsules) and common issues like chronic low back pain can reduce mobility and limit the ability to move efficiently or control the body's center of mass over its base of support.
Chronic obstructive pulmonary disease (COPD)	A loss of normal pulmonary function; results in lower levels of oxygen being placed into the bloodstream. Reduced oxygen levels can affect the ability of muscle cells to efficiently metabolize free fatty acids and glycogen into the adenosine triphosphate (ATP) required to fuel contractions, resulting in lower levels of energy.
Dementia, Alzheimer's, and aging-related cognitive impairment	The aging process can affect the brain in different ways, altering its ability to perform many executive functions, including both short- and long-term memory recall.

Exercise Gives You the Ability to Change How You Age

If you're a certain age, you no doubt know what a flux capacitor is. In the 1985 movie *Back to the Future*, eccentric physicist Doc Brown (played by Christopher Lloyd) famously invented the flux capacitor, making time travel a reality in the fictional context of the movie. It was the flux capacitor that made it possible for Marty McFly (played by Michael J. Fox) to drive a DeLorean sports car into the past; along the way he made sure his parents began a successful courtship and allegedly invented rock and roll. I bring up McFly's trip to the past to make the point that until a real-life Doc Brown invents a legitimate way for us to travel through time, exercise is the only means we have to change how the passage of time affects our bodies.

The good news is that exercise in general, and high-intensity exercise in particular, can act as a flux capacitor, allowing you to retain your youthful strength, power, and aerobic capacity as the years pass on the calendar. The challenge is knowing how to do the right types of exercise in the appropriate amounts to receive the greatest benefits.

Three types of exercise can do the most to mitigate the aging process: mobility training; muscle force production, which includes exercises for both muscular strength and power; and metabolic conditioning with a specific focus on high-intensity interval training (HIIT), which could do more to slow aging than traditional steady-state exercise programs. Yes, we already know that exercise is good for us, and chances are that you already exercise on a regular basis, but up until now most of the information on exercise related to aging has focused on low- to moderate-intensity exercise. If you have already been exercising throughout adulthood, you're used to pushing yourself. You have the ability to function at a high level of fitness and do not need to be relegated to lower-intensity exercise just because of your age.

Not only can high-intensity exercise burn more calories and help create lean muscle, but heavy strength training or explosive power training can produce different responses in the body that may support successful aging. Therefore, you want to be sure to include them in your workout program. You don't have to stop high-intensity exercise as you get older. In fact, this is when it could probably help you the most. You want to make sure that as you age, you exercise not only harder but also smarter.

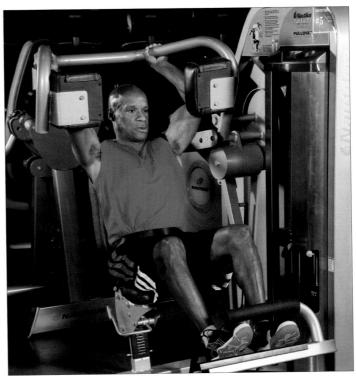

The following sections of this chapter provide a general overview of how the three modes of activity produce benefits that ward off the effects of aging, while the following chapters go into much greater detail. They provide workout programs that could help you not only to burn calories to manage a healthy weight and sculpt muscle to create a favorable appearance but also to retain youthful levels of energy over the coming years.

When combined in a workout program, the three primary modes of exercise—mobility training, muscle force production, and metabolic conditioning—can help slow the effects of the aging process.

How Exercise Supports Successful Aging

All of the systems in the body are made up of cells. One of the greatest benefits of high-intensity exercise is that it results in *mechanotransduction*, which is the process of mechanical forces stimulating the production of new cells in muscle and connective tissues. If your car becomes scratched, you may need to apply some paint to cover up the scratch. As you age, high-intensity exercise creates the mechanical forces that can stimulate production of new cells, which is like carrying touch-up paint to fix damaged tissues in your body. Table 2.4 outlines the systems of the body that receive the greatest benefits from exercise.

Exercise is the essential factor you can use to change how the aging process affects your body. The effects of the aging process can greatly diminish the mechanical, metabolic, hormonal, and neural functions vital for energy production and control of the muscular activity responsible for human movement. Mechanical components of the human body include muscle, fascia, connective tissue, organs, and skeletal structures. Metabolic functions control the breakdown of macronutrients for the production of chemical energy (adenosine triphosphate [ATP]) to fuel muscle contrac-

Table 2.4   **Systems That Receive the Greatest Benefits From Exercise**

Physiological system	Benefits from exercise
Cardiorespiratory	• Improve aerobic efficiency (the ability to transfer oxygen from the air into the blood and circulate it throughout the body)
Neural/CNS	• Increase type II muscle motor unit activation • Improve dynamic balance • Improve nerve conductivity (the ability to maintain quick reflexes and explosive muscle force production)
Muscular	• Improve ability to maintain high levels of force production and mitigate the effects of aging-related muscle loss • Support an efficient resting metabolism • Improve carbohydrate metabolism in the muscle cells
Skeletal and connective tissue	• Increase osteoblast production in order to enhance BMD • Improve joint ROM for better movement • Build stronger connective tissues, more resilient against injury • Enhance production of satellite cells that form new tissues like collagen
Metabolic	• Reduce insulin sensitivity to improve carbohydrate metabolism • Improve anaerobic metabolism
Endocrine	• Increase production of muscle-building hormones (GH, T, and IGF-1)
Cognitive	• Elevate levels of brain-derived neurotrophic factor (BDNF), a protein that can help stimulate growth of brain cells and neural pathways • Improve executive function of brain and memory recall • Stimulate growth of new cells through learning new exercises and movement patterns
Emotional/social	• Improve self-confidence and self-efficacy • Establish and develop relationships with like-minded individuals of all ages through belonging to a fitness facility and taking classes

tions. Hormones are produced in reaction to various stimuli in order to control the functions and actions of specific cells. Neural activity senses an external or internal stimulus and determines an appropriate response.

Table 2.2 on page 22 shows what can happen to the bodies of individuals who remain sedentary throughout the aging process; tables 2.4 and 2.5 feature the benefits from exercise. Comparing the three tables, it's easy to see that the benefits of exercise can address a number of the changes that occur during the aging process. Exercise can't eliminate the effects of aging, but an exercise program that includes workouts for mobility and high-intensity strength and power training in addition to metabolic conditioning can certainly change how aging affects your body. As mentioned, a sedentary lifestyle could result in the loss of between 8 and 10 percent of muscle mass per decade after the age of 40; however, for those who do strength training, that loss can be as little as 2 percent per decade, which is a significant difference (McDonald 2019). The good news is that strength and power training is widely recognized as one of the most powerful means for stimulating muscle growth and can be the most effective way to limit any aging-related muscle loss (Taylor 2013; Fragala et al. 2019; Haff and Triplett 2016; Rice and Keogh 2009).

Table 2.5   **Benefits of Exercise Modes**

Mode of exercise	Benefits
Mobility training	<ul><li>Increase tissue extensibility</li><li>Enhance joint ROM</li><li>Improve ability to perform foundational patterns of movement:<ul><li>- Hip hinge</li><li>- Squat</li><li>- Lunge</li><li>- Push</li><li>- Pull</li><li>- Rotation</li></ul></li><li>Improve dynamic balance (the ability to control a moving center of gravity over a changing base of support)</li></ul>
Strength and power training	<ul><li>Increase muscle size and definition</li><li>Increase BMD</li><li>Enhance resiliency of connective tissues</li><li>Increase production of satellite cells responsible for building new tissues</li><li>Increase production of muscle-building hormones</li><li>Increase muscle force output</li><li>Maintain levels of lean muscle mass for an efficient resting metabolism</li><li>Increase levels of BDNF to reduce risk of developing dementia or Alzheimer's</li><li>Increase activation of type II muscle fibers</li><li>Improve efficiency of glucose metabolism</li><li>Enhance confidence and levels of self-esteem</li><li>Improve functional performance for ADLs</li></ul>
Metabolic conditioning	<ul><li>Enhance cardiac output</li><li>Increase blood flow to muscle tissue</li><li>Increase capillary density</li><li>Increase aerobic capacity</li><li>Enhance mitochondrial density</li><li>Increase energy expenditure (weight loss)</li><li>Lower blood lipid profiles to reduce risk of high cholesterol</li><li>Reduce risk of developing different types of cardiovascular disease</li><li>Increase levels of BDNF and muscle-building hormones</li></ul>

The Role of Mobility Training in Changing How You Age

Mobility is a combination of tissue extensibility (how muscle and connective tissues lengthen and shorten), motor control, and the ability of joints to move unrestricted through their complete ROM. Your body is designed to move; the CNS senses the environment to determine which muscles need to generate force to produce specific patterns of movement. Maintaining optimal mobility could help you avoid many common musculoskeletal injuries associated with aging, like sore knees, a bad back, and achy shoulders.

Muscle contains two distinctly different types of tissue: the contractile element of protein fibers that control force production and the noncontractile element of elastic connective tissues including fascia. Fascia itself has two specific components: (1) the individual protein fibers of collagen and elastin; and (2) the extracellular matrix (ECM), a gelatinous network containing fibroblasts, which are individual cells of fibrous connective tissue and ground substance where proteoglycans hold on to water. The satellite cells that eventually become muscle and elastic connective tissues are formed within the ECM, which plays an integral role in creating the structure of the body. The ECM surrounds individual muscle and fascia fibers like a soft, coarse mesh that contains nerve endings, sensory neurons, and glands responsible for producing specific hormones (Schleip 2017).

One major aging-related change to the human body is that fascia, connective tissues, and ECM retain less water, losing the ability to slide over one another to allow for efficient mobility and increasing the risk of developing adhesions (Schleip 2017). Muscles are organized in layers. When fibroblasts respond to the stresses imposed by poor posture, collagen is produced between the layers; combined with the loss of hydration, the collagen further limits the ability of the layers to slide over one another during movement. The mechanical stress of maintaining poor posture or body position for an extended period of time results in the production of fibroblasts that create collagen fibers to strengthen the affected tissues (Schleip 2015; Myers 2014). In older adults with an excessive forward curvature of the spine (technically called hyperkyphosis), these factors have changed the body to the point where it is stuck in this position, severely restricting mobility of the spine and hips.

Another common issue that can change mobility is performing the same exercise too often. Every joint in the body is surrounded by muscles that produce and control movement. Repeatedly performing the same exercises or spending too much time in a sedentary position could not only lead to adhesions but also cause muscles on one side of a joint to become tight from overuse or lack of use. When the muscles on the other side of the joint lose the ability to contract efficiently, a muscle imbalance could

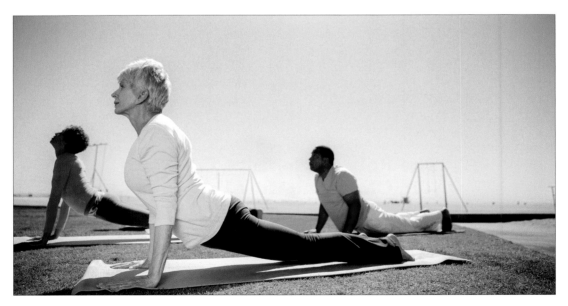

Mobility exercises, like yoga, are essential for ensuring optimal function of muscles, connective tissues, and joint structures throughout the aging process.
Paul Bradbury/Caiaimage/Getty Images

result. Muscle imbalances change joint position; this in turn restricts joint motion and could become a potential cause of injury. A repetitive cycle begins: Adhesions restrict efficient movement, and a lack of movement could result in more adhesions, which could then cause muscle imbalances. For example, a workout program that includes numerous repetitions of the chest press without proper stretching or exercises for the opposing muscle groups can lead to fibroblasts producing new fibers that restrict the ability of the pectoralis major to properly lengthen and shorten, resulting in pain around the shoulder joints.

As you age, maintaining optimal mobility allows you to perform numerous movements without any restrictions that could cause injuries. Mobility-specific workouts that lengthen fascia can apply the tensile forces that ultimately stimulate the production of new fibroblasts for creating new collagen fibers; this helps the tissues to become stronger with a greater capability of withstanding lengthening forces and results in stronger, more injury-resistant connective tissues. Moving a weight such as a dumbbell through multiple planes of motion or simply moving the body in numerous directions through the constant force of gravity results in the production of fibroblasts to increase the strength of tissues that are affected by the mechanical forces (Schleip 2015). Effective dynamic warm-ups before exercise combined with mobility-specific workouts help reduce the risk of developing muscle imbalances, bringing you one step closer to achieving successful aging.

High-Intensity Exercise Creates Overload

Exercise is physical stress applied to the body. Exercise challenges the body to work harder than it is accustomed to, which creates adaptations such as large muscle fibers capable of generating more force and a stronger heart capable of moving more blood per contraction. The principle of progressive overload states that to make the physiological systems of the body function more efficiently, they need to be challenged to work harder than they are capable of. Two primary types of overload create changes to muscle tissue: mechanical and metabolic.

Mechanical overload refers to the physical forces applied directly to the protein structures of muscle fiber. When muscles generate force against an external resistance, muscle fibers can be damaged and must then be repaired. The ECM will produce satellite cells, which are then used to repair the muscle fibers. The result is thicker fibers with a greater cross-width capable of generating higher levels of force (Schoenfeld 2016).

Metabolic overload refers to a muscle working to the point of fatigue, causing the depletion of all available energy. Muscle cells store a finite amount of ATP, the chemical used to create muscle contractions. Muscle can generate ATP either with oxygen (aerobically) or without (anaerobically). Muscle cells will use available glycogen (how carbohydrate is stored in muscle cells) either with or without oxygen to produce ATP at higher intensities of exercise. Exercise to the point of fatigue, indicated by acute muscle soreness or the inability to complete another repetition, will deplete glycogen. During the recovery period after exercise, muscle cells will adapt by storing more glycogen, which holds on to water, causing muscle growth (Schoenfeld 2016). Moderate- to high-intensity exercise programs rely on glycogen metabolism (glycolysis) for ATP; the result of sustained glycolysis is an accumulation of lactate, inorganic phosphates, and hydrogen ions, which elevate blood acidity, a state known as acidosis. Research suggests that there is a strong relationship between acidosis and the anabolic hormones responsible for muscle growth, specifically GH, T, and IGF-1

(Schoenfeld 2016). Even better, there is evidence to suggest a relationship between the high-intensity exercise that results in acidosis and higher levels of BDNF, which in turn helps stimulate growth of new brain cells (Jimenez-Maldonado et al. 2018).

The Role of Strength and Power Training

One consequence of aging is the loss of muscle mass and simultaneous reductions in muscle force output and functional work capacity. Due to factors not yet fully understood, including long-term protein damage and accumulation of ROS, aging-related atrophy will occur even if you do strength training on a regular basis (McDonald 2019). Aging is also related to a slowing of nerve conduction and fiber contractile velocity, resulting in a loss of muscle power (Haff and Triplett 2016).

Strength training is the process of exercising with external resistance to enhance the ability of muscle tissue to generate force, change appearance by increasing muscle size and definition, or a combination of the two. Strength training stimulates specific neural and structural adaptations that can improve the size and force production capacity of skeletal muscle. One effect of a progressively challenging overload is the activation of greater numbers of muscle motor units and the fibers to which they attach (figure 2.2). An appropriately applied overload can improve the neural efficiency at which the muscle communicates with the CNS and lead to an increase in the size or structure of a muscle. Strength training can increase muscle size, minimizing the effects of aging-related atrophy. However, if you're over 40, it's also important to perform exercises that enhance muscle power output in order to improve physical function and retain existing muscle mass.

Strength is the ability of muscle to generate force against an external resistance, while power is the product of force and velocity or the ability to generate more force in a shorter period of time. Strength training and power exercises provide the necessary stimulus to engage and activate the type II motor units and fibers responsible for increased muscle force production. Traditional strength training can help maintain muscle mass, while power training can help that muscle tissue contract more efficiently.

Power training works by changing both the structural and neural components of muscle and can enhance the ability to perform many activities of daily living

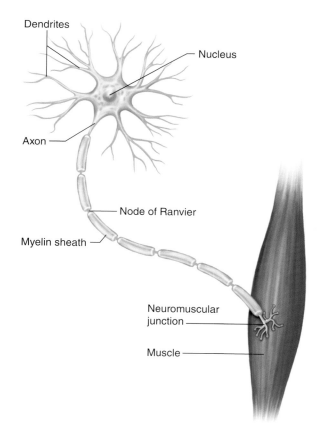

Figure 2.2 By activating numerous motor units, high-intensity strength and power training can help enhance force output in addition to improving energy metabolism. Both help to mitigate how the passage of time affects your muscles.

(ADLs), such as carrying children, navigating a busy urban street, or participating in a favorite recreational activity. Loss of muscle power output is related to loss of ability to perform many physical functions and ADLs; aging-related loss of muscle power is a predictor of falls, motor impairments, and the onset of functional disability (Bet da Rosa Orssatto et al. 2019).

High-intensity strength training and increasing muscle power output can provide greater benefits for improved muscle function than moderate-intensity strength training programs (Fragala et al. 2019; Katula, Rejeski, and Marsh 2008). High-intensity strength and power exercises require the CNS to generate a rapid discharge of motor units; they are most often used for enhancing athletic performance but can also provide many useful benefits for helping you to retain your youthful strength and energy.

The result of a power training program will be that muscle tissue makes both neural adaptations, which change the speed at which contractions occur, and structural adaptations, which promote changes in muscle strength and size. An effective strength and power training program can help minimize the normal physiological effects of the biological aging process, improve quality of life by maintaining functional independence and ability to execute essential ADLs, and be an effective anti-aging benefit (Bet da Rosa Orssatto et al. 2019; Byrne 2016; Fragala et al. 2019). Muscle strength and power are separate attributes that should be trained with specific programs. No matter what other fitness goals you may be working toward, power training exercises can help achieve them as long as you don't have any injuries or muscle imbalances that inhibit skilled movement or limit joint ROM. As you become older, the safe application of power training exercises can be important for successfully managing the aging process.

Even if you have worked out consistently in the past, it is not appropriate to start any exercise program with high intensity. The smartest, safest course of action is to start with basic strength training and gradually increase intensity over the course of three to six months. That may seem like a long time, but it will ensure that your body properly adapts to the stimulus so you can experience the greatest long-term benefits.

How Strength and Power Training Slow Down the Aging Process

Increase type II motor unit activation

Increase speed of muscle contraction

Increase magnitude of force production (ability to generate tension against external resistance)

Improve carbohydrate metabolism (glycogen to ATP) for force production

Enhance strength to perform functional ADLs

Maintain lean muscle mass to slow down aging-related atrophy and sarcopenia (muscle loss)

Increase capillary density for efficient oxygen exchange

Reduce resting heart rate and blood pressure

Increase production of anabolic hormones that promote muscle growth

The Role of Metabolic Conditioning

When it comes to actually driving your muscle car, it is well known that navigating the stop-and-go traffic of a city can burn a lot more gas than sustaining a steady rate of speed on a highway. In addition, the constant starting and stopping of city driving can place much more wear and tear on the systems of a car than highway driving does.

This rough analogy provides an effective insight into how the human body responds to different types of metabolic conditioning, a more appropriate term for what is typically called cardiorespiratory exercise, or cardio (if you're breathing, then technically you're doing cardio). Cardiorespiratory refers to the process of bringing oxygen into the body and placing it into the blood via the lungs and then pumping it to the working muscles via the heart. However, anytime you start exercising, it's your metabolism that actually produces the energy to fuel muscle contractions from one of three different pathways that will be discussed in chapter 7. Because it's one of the metabolic pathways responsible for producing the energy used by muscles for any type of exercise, *metabolic conditioning* is a more appropriate term.

When your muscles are working, they require energy. The carbohydrate, fat, and in some cases protein that you consume are metabolized into ATP in the muscle cells (figure 2.3). When you're at rest (like now when reading this book) or during low-intensity activity, muscle cells metabolize fat with oxygen to produce ATP. When muscles need energy more quickly than fat can provide it, they metabolize ATP from glycogen stored in the muscle cells either with or without oxygen. When muscles need energy *now*, they use existing ATP, which is stored in very finite amounts in the muscle cells. Here's an illustration: When you're walking to a bus stop, you are

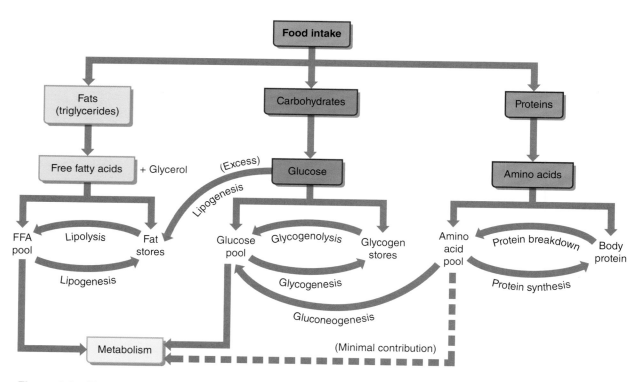

Figure 2.3 The food consumed in your diet is metabolized into the energy used to fuel muscle contractions; fats and carbohydrates are the primary sources of energy with proteins being used only when glycogen is not available.

working at a relatively low intensity, so muscles are producing ATP from fat and oxygen. If you see the bus off in the distance, you may start jogging; as you do, your muscles need energy faster than they can metabolize it from fats, so they will begin to use glycogen stored in the muscle cells. If you notice the bus might arrive at the stop before you do, you may start to sprint, resulting in muscle cells using the limited amount of stored ATP available.

The highest-intensity exercise relies on ATP stored in the muscle cells. Once that is depleted, it must be generated from one of the following sources: fat, specifically free fatty acids are relatively energy dense; a single triglyceride molecule can produce approximately 300 ATP molecules. When glycogen is metabolized in the presence of oxygen, one molecule of glycogen can produce approximately 32 molecules of ATP. When ATP is metabolized from glycogen without oxygen, one molecule yields only three molecules of ATP (Haff and Triplett 2016). The benefit of higher-intensity exercise that relies on anaerobic glycolysis, the process of metabolizing glycogen to ATP without oxygen, is that it is energy expensive; it takes ATP to produce ATP for muscle contraction. This is the reason for the recovery intervals during interval training; these are the periods when your muscle cells are removing metabolic by-product, the "exhaust" from muscle contractions, while producing new ATP for the next interval of exercise. When performing steady-state exercise at lower intensities, muscles consistently use oxygen to help metabolize fats or glycogen into ATP. HIIT, similar to city driving, can be extremely effective for burning calories and improving aerobic capacity but at the expense of placing high levels of physical stress on the body.

Metabolic conditioning at all intensities—low, moderate, and high—can provide numerous benefits to help you achieve successful aging. Lower-intensity exercise can help you expend energy, increase mitochondrial density, and improve the heart's ability to pump blood around the body, while placing a low amount of stress on your body; this is very similar to highway driving in your muscle car. When your body works at a higher intensity, it is burning more fuel because it is using ATP during both the exercise and recovery intervals to fuel muscle contractions and produce more ATP. Benefits of higher-intensity metabolic conditioning include depleting muscle cells of glycogen, which can lead to more efficient carbohydrate metabolism, and muscle growth while creating mechanical damage to the muscle fibers, which stimulates the production of the hormones and satellite cells required to repair those fibers.

How Metabolic Conditioning Slows Down the Aging Process

Expend energy to maintain a healthy weight

Increase levels of muscle-building hormones

Improve carbohydrate metabolism

Improve circulation

Increase cardiac output by improving stroke volume

Maintain cardiorespiratory efficiency

Elevate levels of BDNF to build new brain cells

Anabolic Steroids: The Real-Life Flux Capacitor

The flux capacitor is a fictional structure that makes time travel possible, but in real life it is the anabolic steroids produced by your endocrine system as the result of high-intensity exercise that can help you to achieve successful aging and slow down the effects of time on your body. Anabolic steroids are commonly thought of as performance-enhancing drugs used by athletes. While it is true that some athletes use supplemental steroids to help speed up the postexercise muscle-repair process, it is important to note that anabolic steroids are hormones produced naturally by the human body. High-intensity exercise is an important stimulus responsible for the production of anabolic hormones as well as their associated binding and receptor proteins (Serra et al. 2011; Schoenfeld 2016; Godfrey and Blazevich 2004).

There are two primary types of hormones in the body: peptide and steroid. Peptide hormones interact with receptors on a cell membrane. Steroid hormones interact with receptors in the nucleus of a cell. The term *anabolic* refers to a physiological reaction that promotes cellular growth. (Reactions that break down cells into smaller components are called *catabolic*.) Therefore, anabolic steroids are simply hormones produced by the body to support and promote muscle protein synthesis as well as stimulate the production of the satellite cells responsible for building new muscle tissue (Serra et al. 2011; Schoenfeld 2016).

Just as properly maintaining a car's engine, waxing its paint, and storing it out of the sun can greatly enhance the longevity of its appearance, exercise programs that stimulate the production of anabolic hormones—specifically T, GH, and IGF-1—could help you to maintain your appearance over the course of the aging process. Regular exercise also increases levels of neurotransmitters that facilitate cellular activity, including the catecholamines (epinephrine and norepinephrine) responsible for stimulating energy production as well as BDNF, a protein responsible for initiating the production of new brain cells.

Mechanical Overload and Metabolic Stress Each Stimulate an Anabolic Response From the Endocrine System

Mechanical Overload

Strength and power training exercises use the ATP immediately available in muscle cells in addition to the glycolytic energy pathways while increasing muscle motor unit and fiber activation.

Metabolic Stress

High-intensity exercise increases demand on the adenosine triphosphate and creatine phosphate (ATP-CP) system and glycolytic energy pathways, resulting in an increase in lactic acid and hydrogen ion (H^+) accumulation.

Endocrine System

As the result of high-intensity exercise stimulus, the endocrine system will increase production of anabolic hormones: T, GH, and IGF-1. All play a role in promoting protein synthesis and mediating muscle growth.

The endocrine system will experience both acute and chronic adaptations to exercise. In the acute phase immediately after exercise, the endocrine system will produce elevated levels of T, GH, and IGF-1 to promote repair to the tissue damaged by the exercise stress. Over the long term of an exercise program, the body will experience chronic adaptations of elevated levels of the receptor and binding proteins responsible for promoting cellular interactions with T, GH, and IGF-1 (Serra et al. 2011; Schoenfeld 2016; Goto et al. 2005). Table 2.6 provides an overview of the function of each of these hormones and the factors that influence their production.

In his text on the science of muscle hypertrophy, Schoenfeld (2016) noted that muscle damage as a result of mechanical tension and metabolic stress from high-intensity exercise is an effective stimulus for producing the hormones responsible for cellular repair and that IGF-1 is "probably" the most important hormone for enhancing muscle growth. Likewise, research by Linnam and colleagues (2005) found that "hormonal changes appear to be related to the amount of muscle mass activated and to the metabolic response caused by the exercise."

In their research comparing T production in response to resistance training for three different age groups of men (20 to 26, 38 to 53, and 59 to 72), Baker and

Table 2.6 **Factors Influencing Hormone Production**

Hormone	Description	Function(s)	Factors influencing production
Testosterone (T)	Steroid hormone Produced in: • Males—Leydig cells of the testes • Females—Thecal cells of the ovaries and the adrenal cortex (women produce 10 times less T than men)	Stimulates production of satellite cells, the building blocks of muscle cells Promotes muscle protein synthesis for tissue remodeling (building new muscle cells) Inhibits muscle protein degradation	High-intensity anaerobic exercise that creates acidosis Resistance training: • Large muscle group exercises: deadlift, squat, clean, snatch • High-intensity 85-95% of one-repetition maximum (1RM) • Moderate to high volume (3-5+ sets) • Short rest intervals (30-60 sec) REM cycle of sleep Atrophy of muscle tissue reduces receptor cells and effectiveness of T
Growth hormone (GH)	Peptide hormone Produced in the anterior pituitary gland	Promotes uptake of amino acids into muscle cells and increases the rate of muscle protein synthesis Increases rates of lipolysis (metabolism of free fatty acids for energy) Stimulates release of IGF-1 from liver Enhances function of immune system	High-intensity anaerobic exercise that creates acidosis REM cycle of sleep For women, GH plays a greater role than T in developing lean mass. Resistance training: • Compound exercises • High intensity—10RM • Moderate volume (3+ sets) • 1 min rest intervals
Insulin-like growth factor-1 (IGF-1)	Polypeptide hormone Produced in the liver and muscle tissue	Works with GH to improve muscle protein synthesis and mechanical restructuring of muscle tissue Stimulates satellite cell production	Produced inside individual muscle fibers in response to the mechanical stress that creates cellular disruption or an increase in the amount of GH. The same exercises that increase levels of GH will also stimulate production of IGF-1.

colleagues (2006) found that three sets of six exercises at 80 percent of 1RM with 90-second rest intervals was an effective stimulus to increase T levels in all age groups. The study also found that among all three age groups, individuals with higher levels of lean muscle mass experienced a greater T response to the exercise program. Baker and colleagues noted that an appropriate mechanical or metabolic stress was required to stimulate an anabolic endocrine response and that "older men respond to high-intensity exercise with an increase in T similar to that observed in younger men."

In a similar study comparing the results of the same resistance training program performed by both college-aged (18 to 22 years old) and middle-aged (35 to 50 years old) men, Kersick and colleagues (2009) found that the middle-aged men increased their strength and lean muscle mass while reducing their fat mass at the same rate as the younger men. In addition, the researchers observed that the middle-aged men actually experienced better body composition results than the younger men.

Exercise doesn't just benefit older males; research indicates that women can experience numerous benefits of exercise in their later years as well. In a study comparing the physiological response of women in their 20s and women in their 60s to the same cardiorespiratory exercise program, Ciolac, Brech, and Greve (2010) found that the older women were able to increase their exercise intensity at the same rate as the women almost 40 years younger. Older women can also experience benefits from resistance training and "seem to be able to gain strength to about the same extent as middle-aged or young adults when utilizing a similar type of low volume total body strength training protocol" (Häkkinen 2011).

Rebuilding and restoring an old car to like-new condition requires replacing many worn-out parts and repainting the exterior. While medical technology is now at the point where individual joints like hips or knees can be easily replaced, replacing entire limbs or muscles simply because they get old isn't an option, although that might change in the future as biotechnology evolves. You can, however, gradually progress the intensity of an exercise program to the point where you are using heavy weights for strength training, performing explosive movements for power training, and working to the point of fatigue with high-intensity anaerobic intervals for metabolic conditioning. This could add new muscle, thereby allowing you to improve your appearance in much the same way that a good paint job can help an older car look like new. In their research on how older males respond to resistance training, Izquierdo and colleagues (2001) noted, "Skeletal muscle of older people seems to retain capacity to undergo training-induced hypertrophy when the volume, intensity and duration of the training period are sufficient."

Exercise Can Make You Smarter

One important by-product of exercise for older adults is an increase in BDNF and cognitive function. Exercise creates not only younger-looking muscles but a brain capable of maintaining its optimal performance throughout the aging process (Szuhany, Bugatti, and Otto 2015; Chang and Etnier 2009; Chaddock, Voss, and Kramer 2012; Medina 2017). About their research on the effects of resistance training on cognitive function in older adults, Chang and colleagues (2012) noted: "Our research found that resistance training could positively affect cognition, info processing, attention, memory formation and executive function."

WarGames, the 1983 thriller starring Matthew Broderick as David, a nerd who uses the early version of the Internet to play the first generation of video games, introduced us to the concept of artificial intelligence, where machines are capable of doing the thinking. In the movie, David uses his dial-up modem (remember those?) to search for a computer company so that he can play their latest games before they are released to the public. Instead, he dials into WOPR, a self-learning computer, the early version of artificial intelligence (AI), which was created by the military industrial complex to practice war-game (hence the title of the movie) scenarios about potential conflicts with the former Soviet Union. Instead of playing an innocent video game named "Global Thermonuclear War," David almost accidentally starts World War III when the military thinks the computer simulation is the real thing.

It's amazing how far we have come since *WarGames* was released in the early 1980s; we no longer have dial-up modems and AI has become a reality. You are most likely walking around with an AI machine in your pocket that is more powerful than WOPR, which took up an entire room in the movie. The benefit of AI is that a computer can become "smarter" from the data entered into it; as the computer learns your habits, it can predict what you want when you start typing in a search bar or when it selects ads for a social media feed.

Why this segue into AI? Not only can high-intensity exercise provide health and life-extending benefits, the evidence suggests that it could also enhance your cognitive function. Researchers have identified ways that high-intensity exercise can enhance your brain's performance by producing a protein that helps it and your CNS to work more effectively. That's right, just as playing simulations can make an AI computer like WOPR from *WarGames* smarter, high-intensity exercise produces BDNF, a protein responsible for promoting neurogenesis (the production of new brain cells), which can help improve learning, memory, and other cognitive functions (Jimenez-Maldonado et al. 2018; Church et al. 2016; Voss et al. 2011).

Brain-derived neurotrophic factor is produced primarily in the brain and can help regulate important functions such as creating new circuits for communicating between neurons. In addition, higher levels of BDNF are associated with a lower risk of developing bipolar disorder, schizophrenia, and neurodegenerative diseases like dementia and Alzheimer's. Exercise, specifically the high-intensity exercise that can already slow down the effects of time on your body, can help your brain and nervous system function more efficiently as you get older. As Voss and colleagues (2011) acknowledged in their research review on the topic of exercise and brain function, "There is growing evidence that both aerobic and resistance training are important for maintaining cognitive health in old age."

In the short term, high-intensity exercise can result in greater levels of BDNF compared to moderate- or low-intensity exercise. In a study that compared HIIT at 90 percent of maximum work rate to continuous, steady-state exercise at 70 percent of maximum work rate, the study authors noted, "Shorter bouts of high intensity exercise are slightly more effective than continuous exercise for elevating BDNF." In this study, participants performed an HIIT protocol composed of high-intensity intervals for one minute followed by one minute of rest for 20 minutes, and researchers observed a 37 percent increase in BDNF compared to baseline (Marquez et al. 2015). In a review of the research literature, Jimenez-Maldonado and colleagues (2018) documented that HIIT elevates BDNF after a single session as well as after a consistent program of high-intensity exercise.

High-intensity interval training isn't the only mode of exercise that can affect BDNF levels; resistance training can elevate BDNF both after a single exercise session and over the course of a consistent program. Church and colleagues (2016) compared high-intensity, low-volume (heavy weights, low reps) to low-intensity, high-volume (light weights, high reps) exercise and found that both protocols elevated BDNF, with levels being higher after a single exercise session and at the end of the seven-week study period. "The major findings of this study indicated that BDNF concentrations were significantly elevated after high-intensity, low-volume and low-intensity, high-volume resistance exercise in experienced, resistance-trained men," wrote the authors.

Benedict and colleagues (2013) published results of a brain study of 331 adults who were all 75 years old. The purpose of the study was to understand the effects of physical activity, specifically exercise, on the structure and function of the aging brain. The researchers organized the subjects into four categories ranging from low activity to very high physical activity, and what they found was amazing. They observed that regular exercise slows down the effects of aging on the brain; the brains of the adults who participated in higher levels of physical activity contained a larger mass of gray matter. In addition, the more active adults performed better on cognitive tests and demonstrated more effective memory recall than their less-active peers. This is only one study, and the authors were clear to point out that more work needed to be done to clearly understand the connection between exercise and cognition. However, it adds to the growing body of evidence suggesting that exercise is simply something that must be a part of the aging process to achieve and maintain all facets of optimal health.

Elevating BDNF through exercise could be essential for maintaining optimal brain health throughout the life span; if you exercise for no other reason, it could help you to avoid the cognitive decline that affects millions of older adults every year. The Alzheimer's Association estimates that by the middle of the 21st century, more than 13 million American adults over 65 may be living with Alzheimer's and dementia, costing more than 300 billion dollars annually for health care (Alzheimer's Association 2019) in addition to the devastating amount of emotional and caregiving stress that these diseases place on loved ones. Along with implementing other steps for optimizing brain health during aging as identified by Dr. John Medina in his 2017 book *Brain Rules for Aging Well* (these include participating in continuing education and being actively engaged in a robust social network), adding high-intensity exercise to your regular fitness program could help you to ensure optimal cognitive function well into your later years.

Medina identifies exercise as the "silver bullet" for enhancing cognitive function first because it not only elevates levels of BDNF but also promotes the growth of new blood vessels, which help to bring more oxygen and nutrients to the gray matter. According to Medina, every hard workout could be delaying the deterioration of your brain by as much as 65 days. A second significant benefit of staying active with your exercise program throughout your life span is that it's an opportunity to interact with others, allowing you to develop a robust, real-life social network where you are meeting and establishing friendships with many different types of people, all united by a common interest in exercise. Finally, experimenting with new modes of exercise or techniques for strength training has a component of learning that is critical for strengthening the brain at all ages, but especially in the later years. Learning, whether a new language, a dance move, or an exercise format, can be essential for promoting optimal brain health throughout the aging process (Medina 2017).

PART II

Improve How You Move

3

Mobility and Foundational Movement Patterns

In the original 1984 movie *The Karate Kid*, Mr. Miyagi, played by the late Pat Morita, teaches martial arts to teenager Daniel LaRusso, played by Ralph Macchio. However, before Mr. Miyagi teaches Daniel his particular form of karate, he first requires his student to perform an extensive amount of manual labor, including washing and waxing cars, sanding floors, and painting both the exterior of a house and the surrounding fence. It turns out that the purpose of the chores was to help Daniel learn the necessary motor skills required for practicing karate. In one of the more memorable scenes of the movie, Mr. Miyagi has Daniel demonstrate the movements for "wax on" and "wax off," which turn out to be the techniques required to block the punches of an opponent. One lesson from this classic 1980s movie is that to excel at karate first requires learning the specific movement patterns, like blocking and throwing punches, that determine success. The "wax on, wax off" scene represents the stages of learning and developing a motor skill.

The three stages for learning a new motor skill are cognitive, associative, and autonomous (Schmidt and Wrisberg 2004). The cognitive stage is when you first learn and practice the movement; in this stage, you need to pay attention to specific instructions to make sure you are performing the movement correctly. The second stage, the associative stage, occurs as you are refining and practicing the movement; during this stage, the goal is to rehearse and practice the movement frequently so that you can ultimately perform it automatically as a reflex. The third stage of motor learning, autonomous, has occurred when the movement has become a reflex, capable of being performed without conscious thought. By having Daniel perform hours of repetitive, tedious tasks like washing, waxing, and painting, Mr. Miyagi was accelerating the learning process for Daniel to develop the essential motor skills necessary for success in karate.

The Foundational Skills of Exercise

Just as the moves of "paint the fence" and "wax on" or "wax off" became the foundation for Daniel's karate practice, there are specific movement skills that should become the foundation for a workout program. Your body is designed to move, and efficient movement involves numerous muscles (figure 3.1) and joints working together simultaneously; this is one way to define mobility. Optimal mobility is based on the motor skills and strength to successfully perform the foundational patterns of human movement, specifically the hip hinge, the squat, the lunge (all single-leg movements), the push (forward and overhead), the pull (from the front and overhead), and rotation. Table 3.1 describes each of these movements in more detail; each pattern of movement is visually represented within the table. Performing these movements can help enhance the stability–mobility relationships of joints and muscles; as one set of muscles is contracting to create a movement, the muscles that support that movement are strengthened while the opposing muscles are lengthened to allow the joint motion to occur.

As with karate, once these movement skills are learned, they must be practiced regularly so that they can be performed as a motor reflex capable of occurring without conscious thought. Learning these movements can result in more effective

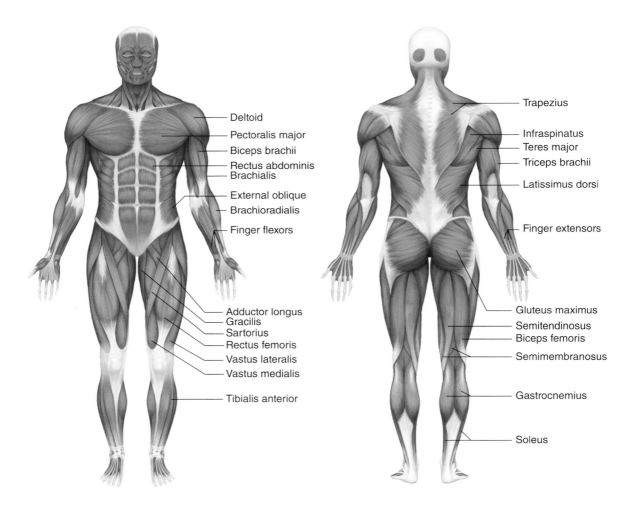

Figure 3.1 Over the course of the aging process, muscles can become smaller and lose the ability to generate significant amounts of force; strength training can significantly slow down aging-related loss of muscle mass.

Table 3.1 **The Six Foundational Patterns of Movement**

Pattern	Muscles involved	Joints involved	Description	Movement mechanics
Hip hinge	Hip flexors (iliacus, psoas major) Hip extensors (gluteus maximus, hamstrings, adductors)	Iliofemoral joints of the hips Intervertebral joints of the lumbar spine Sacroiliac joint	As the glute muscles contract to create the motion of hip extension, the hip flexor muscles are lengthened to allow that motion to occur. The hinge pattern strengthens glutes relative to gravity and can add ROM to the hip joint while maintaining stability of the lumbar spine.	Hinge—bilateral, both feet planted, movement begins from the hips; the knees have only minimal involvement.
Squat	Plantarflexors (gastrocnemius and soleus) Knee flexors (biceps femoris, semitendinosus, semimembranosus) Knee extensors (rectus femoris, vastus lateralis, vastus intermedius, vastus medialis) Hip flexors Hip extensors	Iliofemoral joints of the hips Intervertebral joints of the lumbar spine Sacroiliac joints Tibiofemoral joints of the knees Talocrural joints of the ankles	As the body descends into the squat, the knee and hip extensors and the plantarflexors all lengthen to allow joint motion to occur. As the body rises to the standing position, the hip and knee flexors lengthen to allow the hips and knees to extend. Squat exercises can help establish and maintain optimal mobility of the hip joints while maintaining stability of the lumbar spine.	Squat—bilateral, both feet planted, movement begins from the hips but includes flexion and extension of the knees as well as dorsiflexion and plantarflexion from the ankles.
Single leg/lunge	Plantarflexors Knee flexors Knee extensors Hip flexors Hip extensors Hip abductors (gluteus medius, gluteus minimus)	Iliofemoral joints of the hips Intervertebral joints of the lumbar spine Sacroiliac joints Tibiofemoral joints of the knees Talocrural joints of the ankles	Closed chain triple-joint action in the foot and ankle complex, knee, and hip can improve mobility in hips and ankles at the same time. Unilateral exercise has a crossover benefit—as muscles on one leg are contracting, muscles on the other leg benefit as well. Single-leg exercise should be hip dominant—the initial movement is flexion of the hips prior to motion in the knees; the gluteus medius should contract to create frontal plane stability while on one leg. Because they involve both joints working together, single-leg exercises can help improve hip and ankle mobility.	Lunge or single-leg patterns—unilateral, meaning one leg at a time—may have both feet (e.g., split squat) or just one foot (e.g., one-leg Romanian deadlift) at a time in contact with the ground. Lunges require motion from the hip, knee, and foot and ankle complex all at the same time.

(continued)

Table 3.1   **The Six Foundational Patterns of Movement**   *(continued)*

Pattern	Muscles involved	Joints involved	Description	Movement mechanics
Push	Deep spinal stabilizers Rotator cuffs of shoulders	Intervertebral joints of the spine Glenohumeral joints of the shoulders Radioulnar joints of the elbows Scapulothoracic joints of the shoulders	Push exercises involve stability of the entire spine (cervical, thoracic, and lumbar regions) to allow for optimal mobility from the shoulders. The overhead carry creates stabilization strength of shoulder muscles. The high plank position develops core strength with hands on ground; push-ups become a core strength exercise.	Pushing (forward and overhead)—generating force to move an object away from the body either by pushing forward (or pushing the body away from a solid surface) or directly overhead; requires extension through the thoracic spine, stability of the scapulothoracic joints, and mobility of the glenohumeral joints for optimal motion.
Pull	Deep spinal stabilizers Rotator cuffs of shoulders	Intervertebral joints of the spine Scapulothoracic joints of the shoulders Glenohumeral joints of the shoulders Radioulnar joints of the elbows	Lying supine with arms overhead can lengthen tight back muscles and improve shoulder ROM, making the lying pullover the foundation for the pull exercise before progressing to standing pulls. Standing pulls—using bands or free weights—teach the hips to create stability while the shoulders are working, one of the most effective ways to improve core strength.	Pulling (forward and overhead)—generating force to move an object closer to the body (or move the body closer to a fixed position); requires extension through the thoracic spine, stability of the scapulothoracic joints, and mobility of the glenohumeral joints for optimal motion.
Rotation	Gastrocnemius Adductor magnus Gluteus maximus External obliques Internal obliques Latissimus dorsi	Transverse tarsal joints of the feet Talocrural joints of the ankles Tibiofemoral joints of the knees Iliofemoral joints of the hips Sacroiliac joints Intervertebral segments of the thoracic and cervical spine	The thoracic spine must maintain extension to allow for optimal rotation. When standing, rotation starts in the feet and then moves up through the hips and out through the thoracic spine and arms; the spine remains relatively stable, with the hips providing the motion for rotation.	Rotation—a combination of pulling and pushing; can involve the upper and lower body segments counterrotating relative to one another (for example, the left leg swinging forward, causing the pelvis to rotate to the right, while the right arm swings forward, causing the thoracic spine to rotate to the left).

workouts, which in turn could result in the strength to enjoy the most out of life throughout the aging process. Learning how to hinge from the hips will help you to develop a gluteus maximus that is strong and functional; this is important because this muscle can be considered the power generator for the core. Likewise, learning how to hold a high plank or perform a good push-up can help you to improve your upper body strength while at the same time developing healthy shoulders that allow you to quickly throw your roll-on suitcase into the overhead bin of an airplane.

Exercise for the purpose of enhancing appearance or vanquishing the neighborhood bully may always be important to some of us, but once you get past a certain age, exercise becomes the means for aging successfully. More specifically, mobility exercises become the foundation for using exercise to achieve successful aging. Extensibility is the ability of muscle and elastic connective tissue to lengthen and shorten without restriction. Flexibility is the ability of a joint to move unimpeded through a complete ROM. Mobility is a combination of the two; it refers to the ability to control movement through the complete ROM allowed by a joint. Mobility exercises develop the strength to control joint motion during the foundational patterns of movement.

Developing the strength to control the ROM of these movement patterns is the first step to performing the high-intensity strength, power, and metabolic conditioning workouts that can slow down the aging process. A car designed for performance requires good steering and brakes to control the power of the engine. Producing the strength and power for high-intensity exercise often requires moving from a standing position to generate more power from the ground; therefore, developing good mobility in the ankles, hips, and thoracic spine allows exercise to be performed at a higher intensity for better results.

Muscle and Fascial Tissues

Muscles contain two different types of tissue: (1) the contractile element of actin and myosin crossbridges responsible for producing or reducing force; and (2) fascia, an elastic connective tissue that helps distribute the forces generated by muscle throughout the body (figure 3.2). Within a muscle, the fascia creates the endomysium, perimysium, and epimysium layers, which surround individual muscle fibers, groups of fibers, and the entire muscle, respectively. Striated skeletal muscle is enveloped by fascia and other connective tissues, which when healthy can be pliable, allowing surrounding joints to move easily through their structural ranges of motion (Schleip

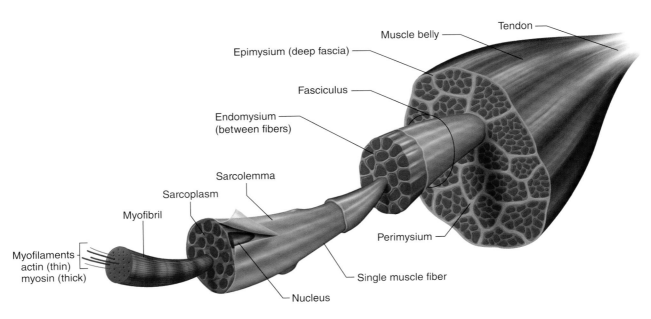

Figure 3.2 Human muscle contains different tissues that perform specific functions; the contractile component of actin and myosin, the smallest units visible, generates force, while the elastic element, specifically the endomysium, perimysium, and epimysium layers of fascia, are responsible for transmitting that force throughout the body.

2015; Myers 2014). However, if a muscle is overused for repetitive motions or held in a specific position during extended periods of inactivity, collagen can form between the layers of skeletal muscle, creating adhesions or knots that restrict the ability of muscle sheaths to slide against one another (MacDonald et al. 2013a).

The muscles, along with their fascia and elastic connective tissues, surrounding a joint function to create movement as well as to provide the stability that controls joint position while motion occurs. Remaining sedentary for extended periods of time and limiting your exercise program to predictable, repetitive movement patterns could result in a significant loss of elasticity, which can greatly reduce the ability of joints to allow mobility or create stability.

Joints do not move on a single, fixed axis of rotation; instead, they experience a constantly changing axis of rotation as a limb articulates through a movement. Optimal mobility allows a joint to experience full, unrestricted motion while controlling the constantly moving axis of rotation. When one part of the body moves, it can influence motion in all other parts of the body. The only tissue that can produce such responsiveness is the fascia that surrounds every muscle fiber. A well-designed exercise program can enhance the elasticity and structural integrity of fascia, restore the ability of muscle tissue to perform multiplanar movements, and allow optimal joint ROM. Optimal mobility and movement skill are based on sensory receptors that upload relevant information to the central nervous system (CNS) about joint position and motion so that it can determine which muscles to activate and how much force to produce.

Fascia can be described as "all collagenous fibrous connective tissues that can be seen as elements of a body-wide tensional force transmission network" (Schleip 2015). Collagen, a structural protein bound in a triple-helix formation to give it rigidity, is produced in response to applied mechanical stress and is used as a building block for many tissues of the body. Fascia is mostly collagen but also contains elastin, a protein that lengthens in response to a tensile (lengthening) force and returns to the original resting position once the force is removed. Collagen and elastin contain fibroblasts, individual cells produced in response to mechanical forces that function as the construction workers of the body because they can repair damaged tissue or build new tissue, including collagen, in response to a mechanical stress. Ground substance is a collection of individual collagen molecules that comprise the extra-cellular matrix (ECM) surrounding individual muscle fibers. The ECM is a viscous fluid that can reduce friction as individual muscle fibers slide against one another. When tissue is warm and moved frequently, the ECM becomes more gel-like, reducing friction and allowing easier movement between individual fibers (Myers 2014).

Injuries related to the loss of joint mobility can be preventable. The ability of fascia to lengthen allows a joint to move through a complete ROM, supporting optimal joint mobility. A lack of motion could cause adhesions between the various layers of muscle that restrict joint motion, which could end up changing the structure and function of a joint. Mobile joints that allow unrestricted movement can reduce stress across the entire system and reduce the risk of injury.

Your body is structurally designed to be energy efficient—specifically, to maximize the use of mechanical energy from the fascia and elastic connective tissue. One important component of improving mobility is doing exercises that have movement in multiple planes of motion to enhance the ability of fascia and elastic connective tissues to lengthen and then return to their original resting position. When muscles contract, they generate force, but it's the fascia that transmits that force throughout the body (Myers 2014). Joints that do not allow a complete ROM could ultimately result in muscles that lose the ability to generate maximal amounts of force.

Mobility Is Required for the Foundational Patterns of Movement

In order for muscles to produce the greatest amount of force, joints should have the freedom to move completely through their structural ROM, which explains why establishing optimal joint mobility is recommended prior to performing the high-intensity exercises that can slow the effects of the aging process. The law of reciprocal inhibition states that as the muscles on one side of a joint contract to move a limb, the muscles on the opposite side have to lengthen to allow that motion to occur. For example, when your biceps shorten to flex your elbow, the triceps on the other side of the joint have to lengthen to allow the elbow to move. In applying the law of reciprocal inhibition, it is easy to see how exercise itself is a form of dynamic mobility. For example, during the glute bridge exercise, as the gluteus maximus muscles (on the posterior side of the hip joint) contract to create hip extension, the hip flexors are required to lengthen to allow that motion to occur.

The foundational patterns of movement involve multiple muscles working together, which requires a balance of stability and mobility. While every joint in the body allows some freedom for mobility or provides structure to create stability, the primary joints that encourage stability are in the knee, intervertebral segments of the lumbar spine, and scapulothoracic area (figure 3.3). The four joints with the greatest freedom for mobility in all three planes of motion (table 3.2) include the foot and ankle complex (actually a number of joints but will be organized into one structure for this discussion), the hip, the intervertebral segments of the thoracic spine (actually a number of separate joints that function together in one unit), and the glenohumeral joint of the shoulder.

The loss of mobility at one joint, even loss of mobility in a single plane of motion, could affect the structure and function of other joints above and below as well as impacting movement throughout the entire body. When a joint's structural ROM results in less movement from the limb, the involved muscles could atrophy and then fail to provide stabilization when needed. Performing foundational movement patterns requires the muscles to control joint motion, and means that they act as excellent mobility exercises. Low-intensity mobility exercises apply the law of reciprocal inhibition to improve joint motion, and can be performed on an almost daily basis to reduce tissue tightness, promote recovery from exercise, and help identify any potential changes to muscle function that could lead to an injury.

How Your Body Learns Movement

A computer is a collection of wires, metal, glass, and plastic. It is possible to go to an electronics store and purchase the hardware to make your own computer, but that computer won't be able to execute any functions without an operating system. The operating system creates the environment for how a computer functions, and software programs, commonly referred to as apps, determine the specific functions a computer is able to perform.

Think of learning an exercise like a hip hinge as downloading the software of a movement pattern; it's this software that activates certain muscles to generate force while telling other muscles to "turn off" so motion can occur. The more often you perform a hip hinge, the more the movement pattern becomes "programmed" in so that when your brain thinks of a hip hinge, it will automatically engage the muscles that need to shorten to produce the movement while relaxing the muscles that need

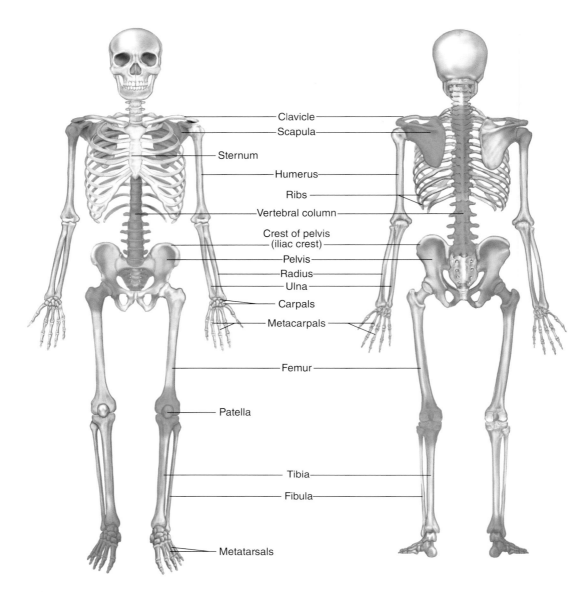

Clavicle
Scapula
Sternum
Humerus
Ribs
Vertebral column
Crest of pelvis
(iliac crest)
Pelvis
Radius
Ulna
Carpals
Metacarpals
Femur
Patella
Tibia
Fibula
Metatarsals

Figure 3.3 A joint is where two different bones connect to one another. The skeleton of the human body contains different kinds of joints; some are designed to provide stability, while others allow for unrestricted mobility. A functional training exercise program to promote successful aging should seek to enhance stability of the stable joints (blue shading)—the knees, the intervertebral segments of the lumbar spine, and the scapulothoracic area—while improving mobility of the mobile joints (red shading)—the foot and ankle complexes, the hips, the intervertebral segments of the thoracic spine, and the glenohumeral joints of the shoulders.

to lengthen in order to allow that movement to occur. In the case of the hip hinge, the abdominals and hip flexors will contract to initiate the movement while the gluteus maximus, spinal erector, and hamstring muscles lengthen to decelerate the forward pull of gravity. If you perform the movement frequently as an exercise, these movements happen automatically.

Your body is like a computer: Muscles, elastic connective tissues, skeletal structures, and organs are the hardware, and the CNS is the operating system that literally brings this hardware to life to control how these parts function as a single, integrated

Table 3.2 **Body Segments Allowing the Greatest Mobility**

Joint(s)	Joint motions	Functional mobility
Foot and ankle complex (talocrural, subtalar, and transverse tarsal joints)	Pronation: combination of dorsiflexion in the sagittal plane, eversion in the frontal plane, and abduction in the transverse plane Supination: combination of plantarflexion in the sagittal plane, inversion in the frontal plane, and adduction in the transverse plane	The foot requires mobility in all three planes when it hits the ground in order to absorb the upward ground reaction forces; as the foot passes under the body, it transitions from pronation to supination to create a stable lever for propulsion. When the foot and ankle complex loses mobility, it creates additional stresses at the knee and hip.
Hip (iliofemoral joint)	Flexion and extension in the sagittal plane Adduction and abduction in the frontal plane Internal and external rotation in the transverse plane	The hip joints require motion in all three planes as they move during the gait cycle. When the right leg is in front of the body, the right hip joint is flexed, adducted, and internally rotated, while the left hip joint is extended, abducted, and externally rotated. If a hip loses mobility in one plane of motion, it could restrict motion in the other two planes as well. In addition, a loss of mobility will affect the joints above (the lumbar spine) and below (the knee).
Thoracic spine (intervertebral segments of the 12 thoracic vertebrae)	Flexion and extension in the sagittal plane Lateral flexion in the frontal plane Rotation in the transverse plane	The motion of the thoracic spine allows the shoulders and arms to work with the legs during the gait cycle; the right leg and left arm will swing forward while the left leg and right arm move backward. This counterrotation helps create the momentum for forward movement. Excessive kyphosis (curvature) in the thoracic spine restricts motion in the sagittal and transverse planes and creates an unstable position for the scapulae. If the scapulae cannot maintain neutral positions, then the motion of the thoracic spine and glenohumeral joints will be affected as well.
Glenohumeral joint (the ball at the head of the humerus connects with the socket created by the glenoid fossa of the scapula)	Flexion and extension in the sagittal plane Abduction and adduction in the frontal plane Internal and external rotation in the transverse plane Abduction and adduction in the transverse plane (when the upper arms are parallel to the ground)	The scapulae create stable platforms for the glenohumeral joints. When the scapulae are out of place, it changes the ability of the shoulders to experience optimal mobility. Improving posture and enhancing strength of the muscles responsible for stabilizing the scapulae can enhance mobility of the glenohumeral joints.

system. Every time you learn a new exercise, you are downloading a new piece of software that controls how the hardware functions. For example, sensory nerves communicate with the CNS about how much muscle force is required and which direction that force should be applied in order to perform a function like blocking a punch or hinging from your hips to pick up a box from the floor. The greatest benefit from the frequent use of consistent mobility exercises is the ability to flawlessly execute the foundational patterns of movement without a single conscious thought. Once your body learns these patterns, the focus of an exercise program should be to enhance the muscular force (strength) you can generate.

Your Body Is Designed for Mobility

Exercise is a function of movement, and the human body is designed to move as one single, integrated system. Walking is a movement that requires almost all of the muscles in the body to work at the same time, albeit while performing different tasks. When we are babies, we learn to walk by simply doing it because the motor pattern is hardwired into the human nervous system. It's necessary to understand the motor skill of walking because it is the default movement pattern of the human body; the muscles and joints of the body are aligned to use the downward mechanical forces created by gravity and ground reaction, an upward force generated as the foot impacts the ground, to help create the energy for forward motion.

The human gait cycle involves the hips and shoulders moving opposite of one another to create the muscular forces to generate forward movement. As you walk, your left arm works with your right leg and vice versa. To use one side of the body as the example, as your right leg and left arm move behind the body, the hip flexor muscles along the front of the thigh and the upper back muscles that connect the arm to the trunk are being lengthened (figure 3.4). Once these muscles shorten, they create the forces to swing the arm and leg forward, which helps propel your body another step toward its intended destination.

Gait requires the hip and shoulder joints, which attach to the bottom and top of the spine, respectively, to function together to produce efficient movement. Compare that to popular isolation exercises, which often only use one part of the body without involving other muscle groups or body parts. For example, a chest press involves only the arm and shoulder muscles; a hamstring curl engages only the muscles of

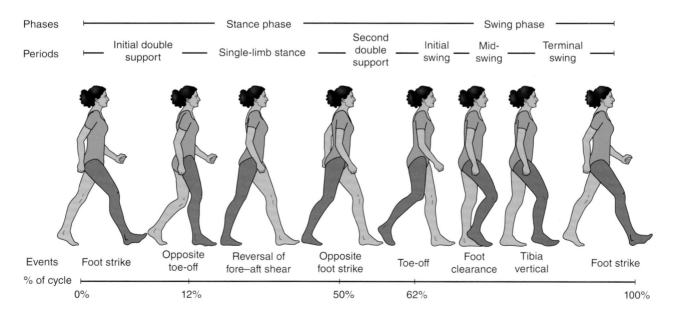

Figure 3.4 The foundational patterns of movement can be seen in the different phases of the human gait cycle: prior to foot strike and midswing—single-leg (lunging) movements; single-limb stance—squatting and hinging; arm swinging forward—push; arm swinging backward—pull; and the chest rotating over the pelvis as the arms and legs perform the different movements—rotation.

Reprinted by permission from E.T. Howley and D.L. Thompson, *Fitness Professional's Handbook*, 6th ed. (Champaign, IL: Human Kinetics, 2012), 60; Adapted from B. Abernethy et al., *Biophysical Foundations of Human Movement*, 3rd ed. (Champaign, IL: Human Kinetics, 2013), 122.

the upper thighs. For optimal movement in gait, the hips need to have freedom of motion that allows one leg to swing forward while the opposite one is moving backward; likewise with the shoulders. Loss of mobility in a shoulder or hip joint not only will affect the muscles immediately around the joint, but can also change how other joints above or below it function.

Gait, whether walking or running, requires multiple muscles to coordinate their actions for successful movement, which is exactly how we should approach exercise. To best develop and maintain strength throughout the aging process, exercise programs should require numerous muscles to work together to produce movement patterns rather than performing a series of separate, discrete actions.

How the Aging Process Affects Mobility

Over the course of the aging process, the tendency is to move less as you get older. However, there is now a population of older fitness enthusiasts who have been exercising throughout their life spans. One thing that these active older adults are learning is that movement itself can often be the best medicine. Arthritis and musculoskeletal injuries like sore low backs or injured shoulders are examples of chronic health conditions that can occur during the aging process, affect your ability to move efficiently, and be a source of frequent pain. Here's a little paradox when it comes to movement: At first it may be a little uncomfortable to move, but once you start moving, your circulation increases, your tissue temperatures increase, and your body releases certain neurotransmitters that dull pain so that it literally becomes more comfortable to move. Yes, there may be minor discomfort when you first start moving as you get older, but if you can tolerate it, as you begin to move you will notice that you feel *and* move a lot better very soon.

As Fragala and colleagues (2019) observed, "For older adults with arthritis, the goal of resistance training programs includes controlling joint pain while improving range of motion, strength and function. Thus, a common barrier to training for individuals with arthritis is the fear of exacerbating joint pain. However, the opposite has been reported, where those with arthritis experience benefit from resistance training without worsening pain or symptoms."

Here's a little insight about strength and mobility: If you do not use it, you will lose it. What happens when a car sits unattended? It falls apart! The same thing happens to your body. If the muscles and joints aren't used in the ways they're designed to, then they could stop functioning properly, leading to a possible injury. However, exercises that move your body in multiple directions can help ensure optimal mobility so that tissues and joints can function when required.

As researchers learn more about how exercise influences the aging process, they are finding that individuals who maintain their fitness demonstrate good physical health and cognitive function, as well. In particular, Berryman and colleagues (2013) observed that older adults who performed better on mobility tests also demonstrated better performance on cognitive tests. Those mobility exercises could be helping to reduce the risk of Alzheimer's or dementia as well as decreasing your back pain.

How Sitting Affects Your Mobility

Whether it is resistance training to build strong muscles, endurance training to improve the ability to sustain a consistent work rate, or being stuck at a desk job for hours at a time, your body adapts to how it is used or, in certain cases, misused. A muscle held in the same position for an extended period of time can change its structure to become shorter. When a muscle does become shorter, it can lose the ability to lengthen when needed, which in turn changes the motion of the joints that the muscle crosses. For example, there is a natural tendency to slouch forward when using a computer while seated at a desk. This changes the length–tension relationships of the muscles around the hips, thoracic spine (upper back, by the shoulder blades), and shoulders.

Sitting for hours at a time results in a posture referred to as upper crossed syndrome. Being in a slouched position can cause the pectoralis major and minor muscles, which control motion of the humerus (upper arm) through the glenohumeral joint, to become tight and restrict a complete ROM. When the pectoralis muscles become shorter, they pull the scapulae forward, which limits the ability of the glenohumeral joint to allow optimal ROM through the shoulder. Losing shoulder mobility could increase the risk of injury from popular activities like swimming, throwing or catching a ball, or swinging a racquet or golf club.

Remaining in a seated position for an extended period of time could cause the hip flexor muscles, which run along the front of the hips to swing the legs forward when walking or running, to become tight and restrict the motion of hip extension (when the leg moves behind the body). If motion for extension does not come from the hip, then it could be generated from the lumbar spine (low back) instead; this could cause a long-term injury.

A bodyweight workout that stretches the hip flexors and strengthens the glutes while improving rotation from both the hips and intervertebral segments of the thoracic spine can mitigate the effects of upper crossed syndrome, helping you to achieve and maintain mobility even if you spend hours a day stuck at a desk.

Mobility Exercises Strengthen Fascia

Like a classic car, muscles function their best when used on a regular basis. If muscles are not used and fibers remain inactive for a period of time, then the collagen molecules of the ECM could bind together for stability; this can create an adhesion between the various layers of muscle. Scar tissue is an example of how collagen produced by the ECM binds together to help a tissue regain its structure after an injury. Once a scar is formed, it can limit the ability of the tissue to move through its normal ROM, which can then affect normal joint function.

During normal movement and activity, collagen will be produced parallel to muscle fibers to provide structure and elasticity, helping the tissue to be more resilient and less susceptible to a strain injury. With a cable machine, a kettlebell, a medicine ball, or a pair of dumbbells, you could perform strength training exercises that move the resistance through multiple planes of motion to help produce additional collagen that allows fascia to become capable of withstanding multidirectional strains (Myers 2014).

When it comes to specific types of exercise, practitioner and author Robert Schleip (2017) identifies the following outcomes required to enhance the optimal performance of fascia:

- Improve extensibility, which is the ability of fascia to lengthen to achieve optimal energy storage capacity for the mechanical energy created during the lengthening phase of muscle action.

Proper Hydration for Connective Tissues Supports Optimal Mobility

Fascia can lose hydration during the aging process, which can restrict the ability of the different layers to slide over one another. Water plays a critical role in lubricating fascia and muscle tissue so that they can achieve optimal levels of function. Because fascia can contain up to 25 percent of the water in the body, it is important to stay hydrated (Schleip 2015).

The ECM component of fascia needs a significant amount of water to allow layers to properly slide during movement. In addition, if the ground substance in the ECM is not properly hydrated, this could slow down the production of new fibroblasts required for tissue repair (Myers 2014). A lack of hydration means that the ECM becomes more viscous and gluey, causing the layers to slide more like Velcro than like layers of frictionless plastic. Improper hydration, combined with remaining in sedentary positions for extended periods, can result in collagen fibers forming adhesions between the layers of fascia. Finally, the amount of water in muscle tissue plays an important role in generating force during strength training exercises. When muscle fibers contract, they push against the fluid in the ECM, creating a hydraulic pressure that adds to the rigidity required for the production of a high magnitude of force (Schleip 2015, 2017).

- Improve the ability of fascia to lengthen in response to applied forces and return to a shortened position once those forces are removed.

- Increase speed of regeneration of fascia after the removal of a strain force to create youthful, wavy architecture of structures capable of handling loads from different directions.

Foam Rollers Can Help Improve Mobility

Referred to as self-myofascial release (SMR), the use of foam rollers for the purpose of reducing muscle tightness has become an accepted component of a workout, with fitness facilities making a wide variety of rollers available for use.

Traditional massage therapy works by manually manipulating muscle tissue to break up collagen adhesions and realign the tissue in order to allow the layers to slide against one another unimpeded. Breaking up adhesions can help reduce muscle tightness and improve joint ROM; however, unless a personal trainer is a properly accredited massage therapist, it is outside of the scope of practice for him or her to apply manual pressure in an effort to break up adhesions. And since it is not practical for the average client to spend the time or money to work with a massage therapist prior to a workout, fitness facilities introduced foam rollers as a means of applying pressure to break up potential collagen adhesions and realign muscle fibers as a component of the warm-up for exercise.

The pressure and motion of a muscle moving on a foam roller can help break up adhesions in muscle and connective tissues, allowing them to function without restrictions (Mauntel, Clark, and Padua 2014). In general, foam rollers provide the greatest response when you place a body part directly on top of the roller and move gently and rhythmically to apply pressure to the underlying tissues. There are two theories about how the use of a foam roller reduces muscle tightness:

1. The first hypothesis on how foam rolling creates length change is based on the principle of autogenic inhibition. This is a natural reflex that occurs when the

Golgi tendon organs (GTOs; sensory receptors located where the muscle and connective tissue attach to bone) detect a change in muscle tension and communicate with the muscle spindles (receptors that lie parallel to muscle fibers) to allow the tissue to lengthen in order to reduce the tension. When a muscle is placed on a foam roller, the tension on the fibers increases, stimulating the GTOs to communicate with the spindles to allow the muscle to lengthen so that the tension is reduced. Note that this is also the basic physiological mechanism for how static stretching creates length change in muscles; holding a muscle in a lengthened position stimulates the GTOs to send a signal that allows the muscle to lengthen (Mauntel, Clark, and Padua 2014; Mohr, Long, and Goad 2014).

2. The second hypothesis about how foam rolling can increase muscle length is as the result of an increase in internal muscle temperature. The friction created by rolling muscle and connective tissue on the foam cylinder increases the temperature of the tissues, allowing them to become more gel-like and resulting in greater extensibility. Once a tissue's internal temperature increases, it is easier to lengthen, allowing surrounding joints to achieve restriction-free ROM (Mauntel, Clark, and Padua 2014; MacDonald et al. 2013b; Healey et al. 2013).

It's not clear which theory is responsible for the outcome, but according to the literature, myofascial foam rolling can lead to increased muscle length, which in turn allows greater joint ROM without loss of strength (Mohr, Long, and Goad 2014; MacDonald et al. 2013b).

Using a foam roller for SMR can reduce muscle tension, which can help lengthen a muscle, but this is a short-term change in the architecture of the tissue (figure 3.5). For best results, it is important to move through a ROM to ensure that the involved tissue can adequately use the change in extensibility and length. For example, if a foam roller on the back of the calf can reduce tightness in the gastrocnemius, then performing a series of bodyweight squats that include closed chain dorsiflexion (how the shin moves forward on the foot during the down phase of the squat) could help improve the functional ROM of the muscles and joints.

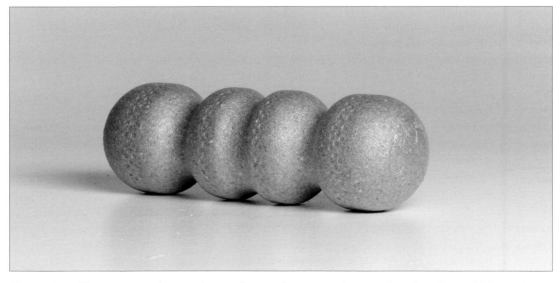

Figure 3.5 The pressure of a muscle on a foam roller causes the muscle to lengthen, which can help improve joint ROM.

The benefits of foam rollers are that they are easy to use and can help provide an acute response for improving muscle length and joint motion; according to published research, using a foam roller for SMR could provide the following benefits (Mauntel, Clark, and Padua 2014; MacDonald et al. 2013b; Healey et al. 2013; Shah and Bhalara 2012):

- Reduce tissue tension, allowing muscles to experience an increase of joint ROM.
- Reduce the risk of developing adhesions from collagen binding between layers of muscle tissue.
- Help reduce soreness after an exercise session, allowing faster recovery.
- Help promote a feeling of relaxation after a workout, an important psychological benefit.

When to Use Foam Rollers

Foam rolling for SMR during a warm-up may help elevate tissue temperature without the use of any exercises that could cause fatigue (Healey et al. 2013). When using a foam roller during a warm-up, it is important to use it only for a brief period to elevate tissue temperature and reduce tension; foam rolling for an extended time could desensitize the muscle, affecting its ability to contract during the workout. Using a foam roller briefly can help prepare the muscles for the mobility exercises that provide the greatest benefit for a preworkout warm-up.

Using a foam roller after the workout, whether as part of the immediate post-workout cool-down or later during the recovery process, could also help to increase the speed of postexercise recovery and minimize the formation of muscle adhesions between layers caused by the natural inflammation that occurs during the tissue repair process combined with a lack of movement after an exercise session. Exercise-induced muscle damage signals the repair process; this is when new collagen molecules are formed to help repair and strengthen tissue. If tissue is not moved, the collagen could bind between layers of muscle. Muscle damage can change the firing patterns of the motor units responsible for muscle contractions as well as change the sequence in which muscles are recruited and engaged to produce a movement (MacDonald et al. 2013a). Foam rolling also offers the important benefit of increasing the feeling of relaxation, which is important for getting a good night's sleep after a hard workout, a key component of postexercise recovery. It would be extremely expensive and impractical to have a live-in massage therapist, but using a foam roller could provide many of the same benefits at a fraction of the cost.

When using a foam roller for SMR the recommendation is to move at a consistent tempo of approximately one inch per second while remaining on areas of tension for up to 90 seconds to allow the tissue to relax and lengthen. Because SMR can help elevate tissue temperature, using a foam roller between strength training exercises could help muscle maintain an elevated temperature during a workout.

MacDonald and colleagues (2013b) conducted a study with two groups: one that used a foam roller after exercise to help reduce muscle tension and one that did not. Their observation was that the foam-rolling group experienced peak muscle soreness 24 hours after a workout while the control group that did not foam roll experienced muscle soreness up to 48 hours after workout. If using a foam roller can help reduce soreness and shorten the recovery time after a workout, it could allow consumers to increase their training volume to maximize results. In another study on the use of foam rolling for recovery, Healey and colleagues (2013) observed, "Post-exercise fatigue after foam rolling was significantly less .... The reduced feeling of fatigue may allow participants to extend acute workout time and volume, which can lead to chronic performance enhancements."

In a review of the research literature undertaken for the purpose of identifying best practices for using foam rolling for SMR, Mauntel, Clark, and Padua (2014) found that applying foam rolling as a component of a warm-up can help reduce muscle tension without limiting a muscle's ability to produce force. A reduction in muscle tension can help improve joint function, allowing optimal movement efficiency and enhanced muscle performance, both of which can help reduce the risk of injury during exercise. The authors observed that gains in joint ROM occurred after only 20 seconds of treatment, with more consistent results being demonstrated after one and a half to three minutes of treatment. "The findings of our review indicate that myofascial release therapies are effective in restoring and increasing joint ROM without having a detrimental effect on muscle activity or performance" (Mauntel, Clark, and Padua 2014).

Foam rolling can be an important component of a preexercise warm-up; it is best to limit the application of pressure to two minutes or less per muscle group. Using a foam roller can help to reduce tension in the tissue; performing a series of multi-planar movements immediately after foam rolling can help develop strength while teaching the muscles to adapt to the new length. One function of foam rolling can be to help reduce muscle tightness before starting the mobility exercises in a dynamic warm-up. For this purpose, use the foam roller for about 30 to 45 seconds on each muscle group to help increase tissue temperature, improve circulation, and reduce tension. Another use of foam rolling is to help prepare for a good night's sleep; a total body foam rolling session in the evening could help reduce muscle tightness, improve circulation, and promote feelings of relaxation, all of which support the exercise recovery provided by a good night's sleep. Table 3.3 provides an example of a foam roller mobility sequence that can be used as a dynamic warm-up or in the evening to promote recovery.

Table 3.3 **Foam Roller Mobility Sequence**

Exercise	Sets*	Time
Foam roller—Calves	1-2 per calf	30-45 sec
Foam roller—Hamstrings and adductors	1-2 per leg	30-45 sec
Foam roller—Quadriceps and hip flexors	1-2 per leg	30-45 sec
Foam roller—Lateral quadriceps	1-2 per leg	30-45 sec
Foam roller—Latissimus dorsi	1-2 per side	30-45 sec
Foam roller—Thoracic spine	1-2	30-45 sec

*When foam rolling prior to a workout, perform only 1 set per muscle group; when foam rolling in the evening, perform 2 sets per muscle group.

Foam Roller—Calves

Benefits

The muscles of the calf are always working; when they become too tight, they can affect mobility at the ankle, which in turn can change how the hip functions. Using a foam roller can help reduce tightness to allow the ankle to have greater mobility; this makes it a great mobility exercise to do before running.

Instructions

1. Sit with your legs stretched out directly in front of you, your hands supporting you under your shoulders, and your spine tall and straight.
2. Place your left calf on top of the foam roller, and bend your right knee so that your right foot is flat on the ground.
3. Move your left calf forward and back to find a spot that is tight or tender (this tender spot is where bundles of muscle fibers have become tight; you will know it when you feel it).
4. Once you find a tender spot, rotate your foot to point toward the midline of the body and then away from the midline of the body. After 15 to 20 seconds, move on to find another tender spot, and repeat for a total of 30 to 45 seconds before switching legs; spend the same amount of time on each leg.

Correct Your Form

To increase pressure on your calf, lift yourself off the ground; if your wrists fatigue, or if the tightness in the calf causes too much soreness, then stay seated on the ground.

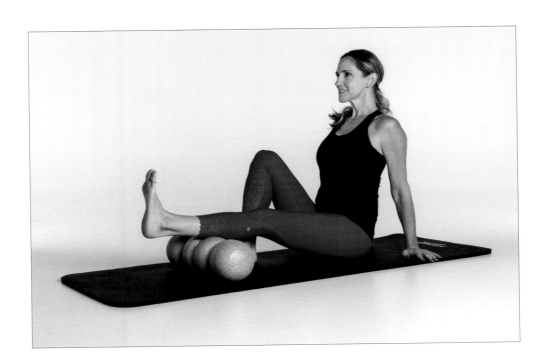

Foam Roller—Hamstrings and Adductors

Benefits

The hamstrings help to extend the hip while controlling motion at the knee, and the adductors work to flex and extend the hip. If either becomes too tight, they can change the position of the pelvis and restrict mobility of the hip joint. Using a foam roller can help reduce tightness to ensure optimal function of the hips.

Instructions

1. Sit with your legs stretched out directly in front of you, your hands supporting you under your shoulders, and your spine tall and straight.
2. Place the back of your left thigh on top of the foam roller, bend your right knee so that your right foot is flat on the ground, and slowly move your leg forward and backward to find a tight or tender spot (this tender spot is where bundles of muscle fibers have become tight; you'll know it when you feel it).
3. Once you find a tender spot, rotate your leg to point your foot toward and away from the midline of your body. After 15 to 20 seconds, move on to find another tender spot, and repeat for a total of 30 to 45 seconds before switching legs; spend the same amount of time on each leg.

Correct Your Form

When your left leg is on the foam roller, use your bent right leg to help support your bodyweight. To increase pressure on your thigh, lift yourself off the ground. If holding yourself off the ground causes too much soreness on the back of the left leg or your wrists, you can remain seated on the ground rather than holding yourself up. It is not uncommon for the muscles on one leg to be tighter than the other, but make sure to spend the same amount of time on each leg.

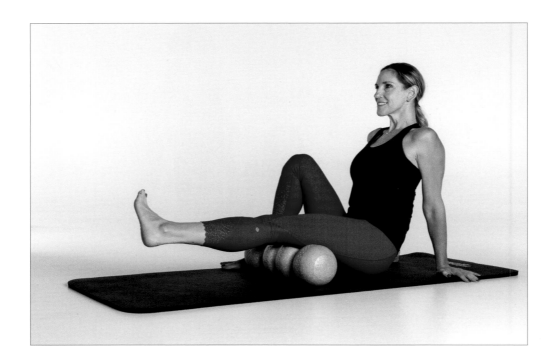

Foam Roller—Quadriceps and Hip Flexors

Benefits

When the quadriceps or hip flexors are too tight, they can create an anterior (forward) tilt of the pelvis, which can change the function of the hip joint. This mobility exercise can reduce the tightness to lengthen the muscles and ensure optimal motion of the hip.

Instructions

1. Lie facedown with your weight supported on your elbows with your legs straightened out behind you.
2. Place the top of your left thigh on the roller, and move forward and back until you locate a tender spot.
3. To increase the pressure, press your elbows into the ground and use your right leg to help support yourself as you lift your trunk off the floor; to reduce the pressure, remain on the ground.
4. Stay on the tender spot for approximately 15 to 20 seconds before moving to the next tender spot; repeat for a total of 30 to 45 seconds, and then switch legs. Spend the same amount of time on each leg.

Correct Your Form

To increase stability, keep your elbows under your shoulders and press them into the floor. If your shoulders start to fatigue, you can remain on the ground to perform the movement.

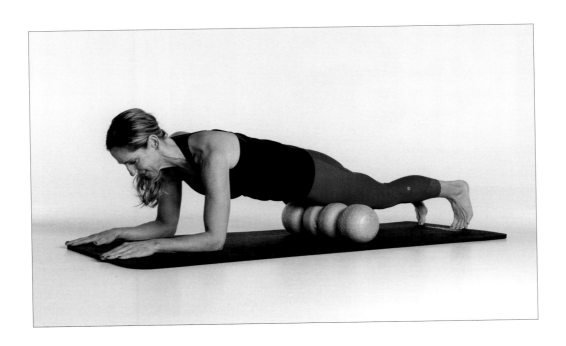

Foam Roller—Lateral Quadriceps

Benefits

The vastus lateralis is the most lateral of the four quadriceps muscles. When it becomes tight, it can pull the knee out of alignment and affect how it functions in relation to the hip. Foam rolling this muscle helps to support optimal biomechanics of the lower body.

Instructions

1. Lie on your right side with your right elbow directly under your right shoulder. Start with the foam roller under the right thigh, just above the knee.
2. Supporting your bodyweight with your elbow, cross your left leg over the right to place your left foot on the floor.
3. Slowly roll up and down the outside of your right thigh. When you find a tight spot, stay there for 5 to 10 seconds to help reduce the tightness; repeat for a total of 30 to 45 seconds. Spend the same amount of time on each leg.

Correct Your Form

To decrease the pressure on the muscles of your thigh, support more of your bodyweight with your left leg by pressing your left foot into the floor. To increase the pressure and the stretch effect, place your left leg on top of the right and support your bodyweight with only your elbow.

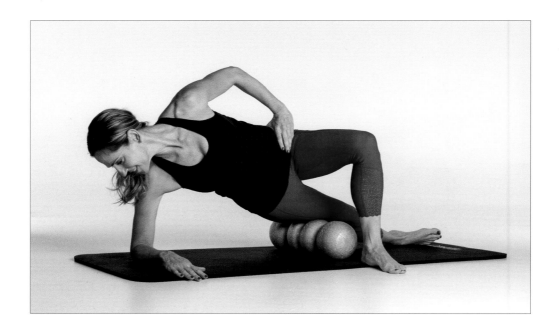

Foam Roller—Latissimus Dorsi

Benefits

The large latissimus dorsi muscle of the back can create internal rotation at the glenohumeral joint of the shoulder; when the muscle is too tight, it can pull your shoulders forward, which can cause back pain. This mobility exercise can help restore and maintain optimal mobility at the shoulder joint.

Instructions

1. Lie on your right side with your right arm lengthened overhead and the foam roller underneath it close to your armpit.
2. Slowly roll in the direction of your hand. When you find a tight spot, stay on it, and slowly roll toward and then away from the front of your body for 15 to 20 seconds; then move to another tender spot on the muscle.
3. Repeat for a total of 30 to 45 seconds before switching sides of the body; spend the same amount of time on each side.

Correct Your Form

Keep your arm extended straight overhead to make sure you can find a tight or tender spot. Use your left hand to help support your bodyweight.

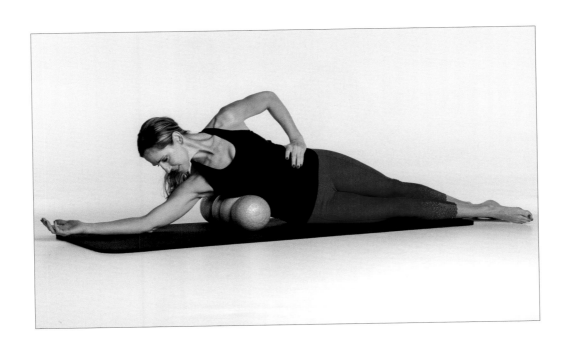

Foam Roller—Thoracic Spine

Benefits

This mobility exercise can help reduce tightness of the erector spinae muscles that run along the spine; when these muscles become too tight, they can restrict motion of the intervertebral segments of the thoracic spine. Reducing tightness in these muscles can help to ensure optimal motion of the upper back. This is an excellent mobility exercise for when you've been seated all day and your upper back is a little sore.

Instructions

1. Place the roller under your upper back as you lie on your back with your legs bent and your feet flat on the floor to help support your bodyweight.
2. Slowly roll toward and away from your feet. When you find a tender or tight spot, stay on it for 15 to 20 seconds while slowly flexing (*a*) and extending (*b*) your spine before moving to find another tight spot.
3. Repeat for a total of 30 to 45 seconds.

Correct Your Form

If it's difficult to support your bodyweight with your legs, place your tailbone on the ground. If the hamstring muscles along the back of your legs start cramping, move your feet away from your tailbone.

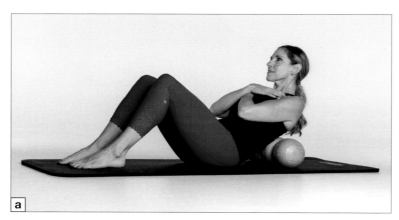

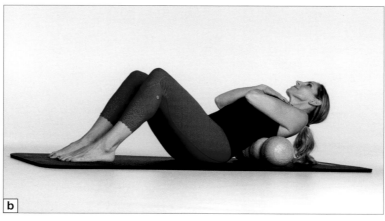

Selecting a Foam Roller for Your Needs

When the use of foam rollers for SMR was introduced, it was such a new concept that there were only a limited number of options available for use. As foam rolling has become an accepted fitness practice, a wide variety of rollers has been created, each promoting specific benefits. Table 3.4 provides an overview of the types of equipment for SMR and their primary advantages and disadvantages.

Table 3.4 **Types of Equipment for SMR and Their Benefits**

Type	Description	Advantages	Disadvantages
Soft core foam roller	These rollers are made of soft foam that is easier to compress, placing less force directly on the muscle.	The pliable surface allows greater contact with muscle tissue. May be more comfortable when first starting foam rolling.	Over time, repeated use can cause foam to change shape and become compressed, reducing its effectiveness. May not apply enough force for extremely active and fit individuals.
Hard core foam roller	These rollers have an outer surface of foam and an inner core made from hard plastic.	Will maintain shape over repeated uses. Can apply a significant amount of pressure to the area of muscle contact.	May apply too much pressure and cause discomfort for some individuals.
High-density foam roller	These rollers are made from specific types of dense foam that is more resistant to compression.	The density allows greater pressure to be placed on areas of adhesion and tightness. The thicker foam allows the roller to maintain its shape longer. These are an option for individuals who may not experience benefits from a soft roller but are not yet ready for a roller with a hard inner core.	May be too dense and cause discomfort for some individuals.
Foam roller with patterns or grooves	These rollers have a specific pattern or grooves that place pressure on different parts of a muscle.	Applying different amounts of pressure on different parts of a muscle may promote circulation.	Depending on the type of roller, the patterning could cause increased pressure in certain areas, leading to discomfort.
Ball	The spherical shape of a ball allows pressure to be focused on specific areas. Like foam rollers, these can come in a variety of sizes and densities. Many companies make specific SMR balls, but almost any ball (e.g., golf, tennis, lacrosse, or inflatable) can be used.	The density and size of the ball allows pressure to be placed directly on specific areas of the muscle.	The surface of the ball may be difficult to apply to a targeted area of adhesion. Certain balls may be too dense and cause discomfort or pain.
Rolling stick	This is a handheld device that can be used to apply pressure and create friction directly on adhesions and areas of tightness.	Allows force to be applied directly to an adhesion or area of discomfort.	Can be hard to use on certain areas of the body.

4

Mobility Exercises and Workouts

As we age, it's no longer enough to simply hold muscles in lengthened position and "stretch" them for 30 seconds; we have to learn how to control our bodies through space so we can stretch, lengthen, and strengthen muscles the way they actually function. Practicing mobility can help you to become more mobile. Mobility workouts are an important component of your overall workout program. Exercise is physical stress imposed upon the body; when your body is sore from a high-intensity strength, power, or metabolic conditioning workout, a low-intensity mobility workout where you move your muscles and joints through multiple planes of motion can help increase oxygen flow and be the perfect recharge to boost your energy.

You can improve mobility and strengthen fascia with a variety of movements in multiple directions, at multiple speeds, and reaching your hands to different heights to add length to the tissues. You should engage in proper fascia loading to improve strength, specifically the ability to withstand tensile forces, two to three days per week, while allowing at least 24 to 48 hours between workouts for fibroblasts to repair and build new collagen (Schleip 2017).

The following are a few points to remember about exercises to strengthen fascia and elastic connective tissues:

- Start with small movements with a limited range of motion (ROM) and gradually build up tolerance for strain through increased ROM and movement speed.

- As with all other exercises, begin with a low rep range to limit the amount of stress imposed upon the tissue; as the fascia adapts to the loads, gradually increase the number of repetitions.

- Remain hydrated to allow for optimal energy storage. The extracellular matrix (ECM) surrounding the fascia contains water, which is necessary for optimal function of the tissue as the layers slide over one another.

- Exercises that move the arms and legs in opposite directions can use specific lines of pull through the fascia to increase length and tensile strength.

Improving mobility in the hips and upper back can reduce overall muscle tightness while improving mobility throughout the body. The mobility workouts in this chapter, which focus primarily on moves for the hips and thoracic spine, have three levels of progression. The first level of mobility exercises takes place supported by the floor; this reduces the effect of gravity for work on joint position and muscle length. The second level of mobility exercises takes place in a standing position. The third level of mobility exercises focuses on dynamic movement between the hips and shoulders; this both improves overall mobility and engages balance reflexes to enhance overall muscle function. The third level of mobility exercises provides a great option for days when you might need to recover from a high-intensity workout the day before. Each of the mobility workouts that follow can be performed as a dynamic warm-up prior to a resistance training workout program or as an active recovery workout. When using one of these mobility workouts for a dynamic warm-up, perform one to two sets of each exercise; when using a mobility workout as a stand-alone workout on an active recovery day, do three to four sets of each exercise.

Supported Mobility Exercises

Lying on the ground in either a supine (faceup; you can remember because the second and third letters spell "up") or a prone (facedown) position reduces the influence of gravity to allow more motion from the hips and thoracic spine. When the body is upright, gravity pulls it straight down, compressing the joints of the thoracic spine and hips; gravity could also pull the upper body forward, causing the spine to have more curvature, which restricts mobility. Lying on the ground removes vertical compression from gravity; this allows the spine to fully extend, resulting in greater mobility for the hips and shoulders. Table 4.1 provides a sequence of ground-based mobility exercises to improve hip and shoulder mobility.

Table 4.1 **Ground-Based Mobility Exercise Sequence**

Exercise	Sets	Repetitions/time
Child's pose cross-body reach	2 per side	30-45 sec hold
Supine hip circles	2	8-12 circles in each direction, first with both legs together, then with each leg individually
Supine hip crossover (L-stretch)	2-3 per side	30-45 sec hold
Upward-facing dog	2	30-45 sec hold
Kneeling offset adductor stretch with trunk rotation	2 per side	5-6 rotations in 30-45 sec
High plank Spiderman with reach to rotation	2 per side	5-6 rotations
Hip rotation to kneeling	2	4-5 to each side

Child's Pose Cross-Body Reach

Benefits

This mobility exercise reduces tension and tightness in the upper back muscles to increase ROM of the shoulder joints.

Instructions

1. Kneel with your feet tucked under your body. As you lower your bottom toward your heels, reach your left arm across your body and over your right arm with the palm of your left hand facing up.
2. Look to the right as you sink your weight back into your hips. Hold for 30 to 45 seconds. Repeat with the right arm.

Correct Your Form

While in the kneeling position, allow your legs to spread open slightly so that your trunk lowers between your thighs. Exhale as you sink back to increase the stretch.

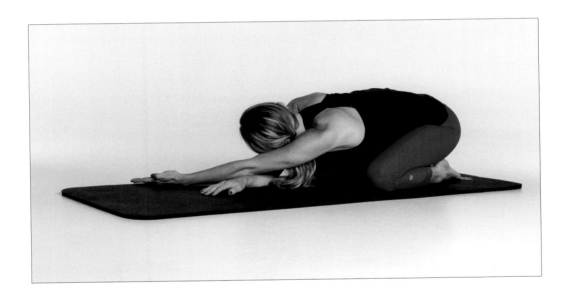

Supine Hip Circles

Benefits

Lying down reduces the effect of gravity. The spine is in a neutral position, supported by the ground, which can increase the available ROM in the hip joints. This mobility exercise can increase tissue temperature and fluid in the hip joint capsules. Mobilizing one hip while keeping the other hip stable can improve mobility in each joint. This movement is a great opener after spending an excessive amount of time in a seated position.

Instructions

1. Lie flat on your back, then bend the knees so that your feet are closer to your tailbone. Place your right hand on your right knee and your left hand on your left knee as you pull both knees closer to your chest.

2. Circle both knees by pulling them up to your chest and then pulling your right knee out to your right side and left knee out to your left side so that both knees are moving away from the midline of your body. Perform 8 to 12 circles in this direction; then perform 8 to 12 circles in the opposite direction, starting from the outside of the body and moving toward the midline and down away from your trunk.

3. Hold the right knee stable, and with the left hand on the left knee, circle the left hip 8 to 12 repetitions in each direction—both clockwise and counterclockwise. Then switch hips—hold the right hand on the right knee, and circle the right hip for 8 to 12 repetitions in each direction.

Correct Your Form

Keep your low back on the ground while moving your hips. Allow your head to rest comfortably on the ground so that your spine remains in an extended position.

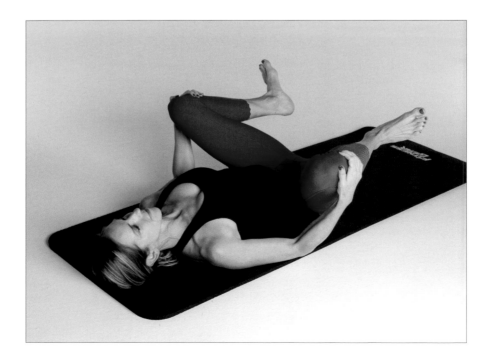

Supine Hip Crossover (L-Stretch)

Benefits

This exercise improves mobility and ROM of the thoracic spine and oblique muscles that control trunk rotation. It also reduces tightness in the muscles that cause external rotation of the hip while stretching the shoulder and chest muscles.

Instructions

1. Lie on your back with your right arm extended straight out to the right, palm up. Keeping your left leg straight, bend your right leg at the hip and knee and cross your right leg over your left so that your right knee is pointing toward the left side of your body at nine o'clock.
2. Place your left hand on your right knee, and press it toward the ground while looking down your right arm.
3. To increase the stretch, press your right knee up into your left hand, hold the contraction for 3 to 5 seconds, and then relax and move the knee down into a deeper ROM. Hold the stretch for 30 to 45 seconds, repeating the contraction 3 to 4 times.
4. Rest briefly, and repeat on the other side.

Correct Your Form

Keep your left leg straight as you cross your right leg over it. Press your extended arm (the right arm in the instructions) into the floor to increase the stretch. Breathe normally; on the exhale, increase the stretch by increasing the pressure of your left hand on your right knee. For best results, keep looking down your extended arm while pressing on the top of the knee.

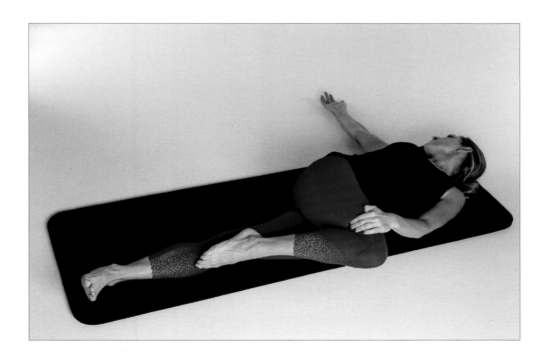

Upward-Facing Dog

Benefits

Remaining in a seated position for too long can cause the hip flexors, quadriceps, and abdominal muscles to become tight and restrict motion at the hips and low back. This move can help lengthen the muscles along the front of your body to ensure optimal posture and motion of the hip joints.

Instructions

1. Lie prone (facedown) on the ground with your legs extended, your hands directly under your shoulders, your upper arms next to your rib cage, and your elbows pointed toward your feet.
2. Press your hands into the ground to lift your chest and thighs off the ground, creating full extension of the spine.
3. To increase the intensity of the stretch, squeeze your glutes while pressing your hips down. Hold for 30 to 45 seconds before lowering to the ground.

Correct Your Form

Only go to a comfortable ROM; do not try to force a backward bend of the spine. If holding your entire body is too challenging for you, practice lifting only your chest off the ground.

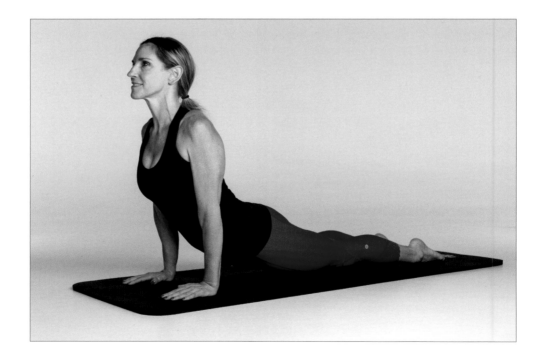

Kneeling Offset Adductor Stretch With Trunk Rotation

Benefits

This exercise stretches and lengthens the hip flexor and adductor muscles, which can reduce tightness in the lower back while improving mobility of the hips.

Instructions

1. Start in a kneeling position with your left knee directly under your left hip and your right foot on the floor. Turn your right leg so that it is pointing 90 degrees to the right (if the left hip is at twelve o'clock, the right knee should be pointing toward three o'clock).

2. Press your left knee into the ground as you lean your weight into your right leg (think about trying to create distance between your right hip and left knee). Hold the end ROM for 4 to 6 seconds, and slowly return to the starting position.

3. To increase the stretch, at the end of the movement, use your right arm to reach across your body, rotating your shoulders and upper back to your left.

4. Slowly move in and out of the stretch, and then switch sides; you should aim to perform 5 to 6 reps in 30 to 45 seconds.

Correct Your Form

Open the hips wide; the right thigh should be at approximately 90 degrees relative to the left. Press the left knee into the floor to increase the stretch on the adductor muscles of the inner thigh. Keep your spine straight while rotating; lift the chest and pull the shoulders back to maintain proper length in your spine. To increase the rotation of your spine, pull back with your left elbow as you reach across your body with your right arm.

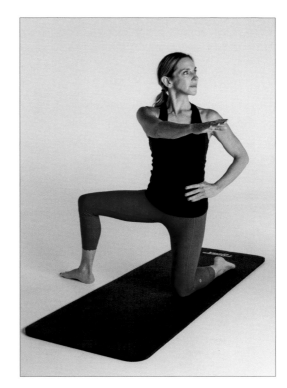

High Plank Spiderman With Reach to Rotation

Benefits

This exercise improves mobility of both the hips and thoracic spine while strengthening the deep core muscles responsible for stabilizing the lumbar spine and pelvis.

Instructions

1. Start in a high plank position with your hands a little wider than your shoulders and feet in line with the hips (*a*).
2. Bring your left knee forward to the outside of your left elbow while pushing back through your right heel to straighten your right leg and increase the stretch of your hip flexors.
3. Pause for 3 to 4 seconds; then use your left arm to reach under your right shoulder (*b*) before rotating to your left and reaching up in the air (*c*).
4. Keep your right hand pressed into the ground and slowly move your left arm to perform 5 to 6 reps before switching legs and repeating with the other arm.

Correct Your Form

Keep your spine straight, and press your hands into the floor to engage the deep core muscles while slowly rotating your shoulders and thoracic spine. Exhale while reaching under the opposite arm, and inhale as you reach up with your arm.

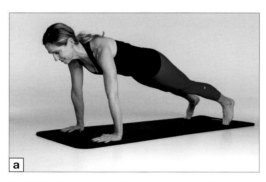

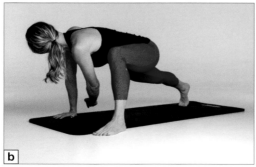

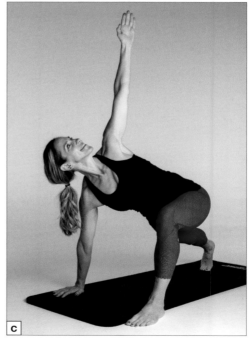

Hip Rotation to Kneeling

Benefits

This challenging mobility exercise uses movement in multiple directions to ensure an optimal stretch of the muscles that control the motion of the hips. Squeezing the glute muscles on your kneeling leg while pressing the hip forward can lengthen the hip flexor muscles, which often become tight from too much sitting.

Instructions

1. Sit on the ground with your legs bent, your feet directly in front of you, your knees pointed toward the ceiling, and your spine in a tall and lengthened position (a).
2. Keep your hands in front of your body as you drop both knees to the left side of your body (b). As the outside of your left thigh touches the floor, push your left thigh into the ground and swing your right leg toward the left side of your body (c).
3. The goal is to finish in a kneeling position, facing in the opposite direction from where you started, with your left knee directly under your left hip and your right foot flat on the ground in front of your body. Squeeze the glute muscles on your left side while pushing your left leg forward to increase the stretch.
4. To return to the original position, pick up your right foot and bring your right leg back closer to your body as you place the inside of the right knee on the ground in front of your hips before rotating back to a seated position with your feet flat on the floor. Alternate sides for a total of 4 to 5 reps on each.

Correct Your Form

Making the transition from being seated with the outside of the left thigh and the inside of the right on the ground to kneeling can be tough. If it is too challenging, start learning the movement by simply dropping both knees to the floor to your left and then rotating them back to the right side of your body.

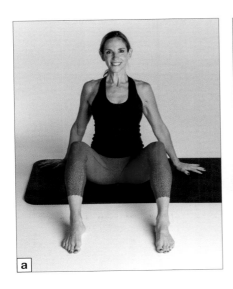
a

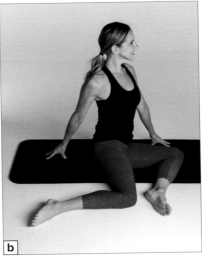
b

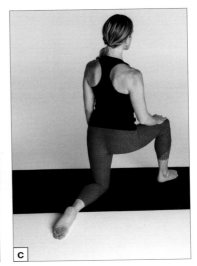
c

Standing Mobility Exercises

The human body is designed to move from a standing position, so standing for mobility exercises allows you to move tissues and joints the way they normally function during upright movements. Stretching the ankle, hip, and shoulders at the same time while in a standing position can help reduce muscle tightness and improve joint motion, which is important for achieving pain-free movement. Integrating upper and lower body muscles into the same movement can help reduce muscle tightness while improving overall mobility. These standing mobility exercises could be performed as a dynamic warm-up prior to a strength training or metabolic conditioning workout or as a stand-alone workout to help promote recovery from a hard workout when muscles are still sore. When performing the exercises as a warm-up, complete one to two sets of each exercise; for a stand-alone workout, complete three to four sets of each exercise. Table 4.2 provides a sequence of standing mobility exercises to improve joint motion and reduce tightness.

Table 4.2 **Standing Mobility Exercise Sequence**

Exercise	Sets	Repetitions/time
Neck stretch	2	30-45 sec hold each side
Chest stretch	2	4-6 with 5-7 sec hold
Type 2 thoracic mobility	2	10-12 each side with 1-2 sec hold
Split stance with one-arm overhead reach	2	10-12 each arm
Standing hamstring stretch with rotation	2	8-10 rotations in 30-45 sec per leg
Calf stretch with rotation	2	8-10 rotations to each side with 1-2 sec hold per leg
Wide adductor stretch	2	30-45 sec hold each side

Neck Stretch

Benefits

Leaning your head forward to look at a mobile device or a computer screen can fatigue the neck muscles, making them tight. This stretch can help reduce that tightness to ensure optimal mobility of the cervical spine.

Instructions

1. Stand with your feet shoulder-width apart and spine fully extended.
2. Drop your right ear directly toward your right shoulder while at the same time externally rotating your left shoulder (so the palm of your left hand is facing forward).
3. When you reach the end ROM, rotate your head to look toward your right shoulder and place your right hand on the left side of your chin. Gently press on the left side of your chin while holding the stretch for 30 to 45 seconds. Switch sides.

Correct Your Form

Lean your head directly to the side; if it moves forward before you drop your ear toward your right shoulder, the stretch could cause additional strain along your cervical spine. Creating external rotation of the left shoulder while rotating to look toward your right shoulder can increase the stretch of the muscles along the left side of your neck.

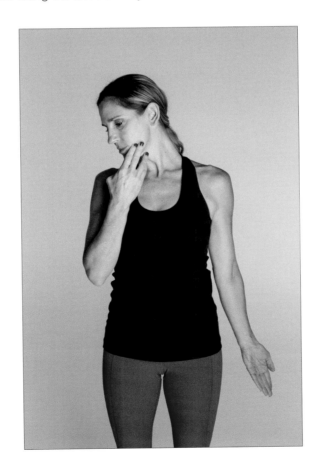

Chest Stretch

Benefits

The large muscles of the chest cause internal rotation at the shoulder joints. When they become tight, they can cause discomfort in the neck and upper back; stretching these muscles can relieve tension and tightness in your upper back and neck while improving mobility of your shoulders. Contracting the muscles of the upper back (pulling your shoulders back) can help release and lengthen tight chest and shoulder muscles.

Instructions

1. Stand with your feet shoulder-width apart, and place both hands behind your head with your elbows pointed directly out to the side.
2. Press your feet into the ground as you squeeze your glutes while lifting your chest and pulling your elbows back.
3. Breathing comfortably, hold your elbows back for 5 to 7 seconds, relax for 1 to 2 seconds, and then repeat 4 to 6 times.

Correct Your Form

To achieve an optimal stretch along the front of your shoulders, make sure you are standing tall and your spine is long. In addition, pressing your feet into the floor while contracting your glutes can help to release the muscles along the front of your body.

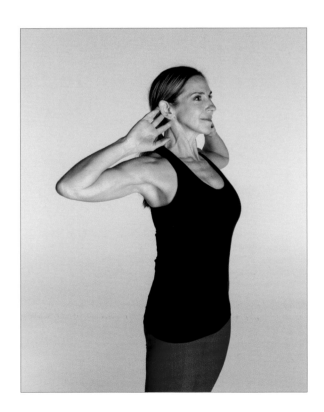

Type 2 Thoracic Mobility

Benefits

This movement uses lateral flexion and rotation to create spinal motion in two different planes (frontal and transverse), which can help reduce tightness of the muscles while increasing mobility of the intervertebral joints of the thoracic spine.

Instructions

1. Stand tall with your feet shoulder-width apart, your knees slightly bent, and your spine fully extended. Raise your right arm to reach over the top of your head toward the left side of your body (as if shooting a hook shot in basketball) so that your trunk leans to the left (*a*).
2. While your right arm is reaching over the top of your head, use your left arm to reach across the front of your body toward three o'clock, causing your shoulders to rotate to your right (*b*). The result should be that your upper body is leaning to the left while rotating to your right. Hold briefly, no more than 1 to 2 seconds for each repetition. Complete 10 to 12 repetitions before switching arms and directions.

Correct Your Form

For optimal mobility through the joints, start with a tall, straight spine. As your arm reaches across your body, allow your trunk and shoulders to rotate to the other side to create optimal motion in the spine.

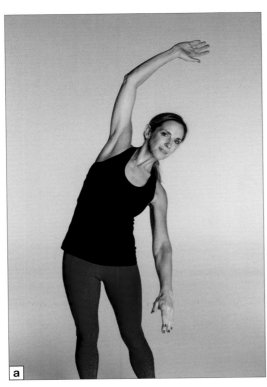

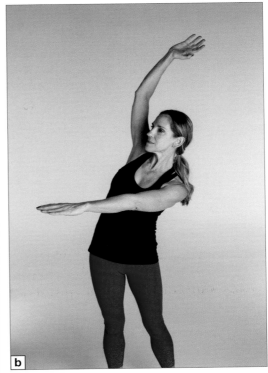

Split Stance With One-Arm Overhead Reach

Benefits

The hip flexor muscles along the front of your hip can become tight from too much sitting, which can reduce the ROM of the hip joint while affecting the ability of the glute muscles to extend your hip. This stretch lengthens the large hip flexor muscles from both the bottom and the top to allow for optimal mobility of the hip and function from the glutes. In addition, this move helps to lengthen the large latissimus dorsi muscles of the back to help improve shoulder mobility.

Instructions

1. Stand with your feet hip-width apart, extend your right leg behind you, and press your right heel into the ground while maintaining a level pelvis.
2. Extend your right arm overhead with your palm facing the midline of your body.
3. Keep your right arm extended and your right heel pressed into the ground, as you reach the right arm behind your head in slow, rhythmic movements.
4. Perform about 10 to 12 repetitions of reaching behind you, and then switch sides. Do the same number of reps on each side of the body. For an additional stretch, squeeze the glutes of the extended leg.

Correct Your Form

For an optimal stretch of the hip flexors, keep the heel of your back foot pressed into the ground while your arm reaches behind you. Keep your spine long throughout the stretch.

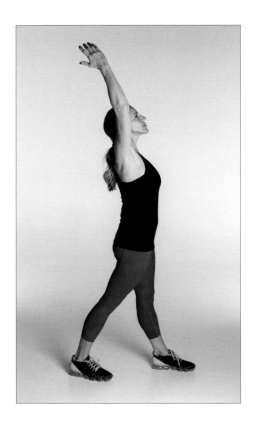

Standing Hamstring Stretch With Rotation

Benefits

There are three different hamstring muscles: two running along the inside of your thigh (medial) and one running along the outside (lateral). Extending your leg lengthens all three hamstring muscles in the sagittal plane, while rotating your leg from side to side lengthens the hamstring muscles in the transverse plane. Dynamically stretching the hamstrings prior to exercise helps to ensure that your glute muscles work efficiently to control motion at the hip.

Instructions

1. From a standing position, straighten your right leg directly in front of you, heel on the ground and toes pointing up, while pushing your hips back and placing both hands on your bent left thigh.
2. Keeping your weight shifted back into your hips, rotate your right foot to point toward the midline of your body and then away from the midline of your body.
3. Hold the stretch for 30 to 45 seconds while slowly moving the foot to perform 8 to 10 rotations. Switch legs and repeat, making sure to do the same number of reps with each leg.

Correct Your Form

For an optimal stretch, keep your forward leg (the right in the instructions) straight throughout the stretch. Rotate the leg slowly, and as you feel the stretch increase, push your weight farther back into your hips.

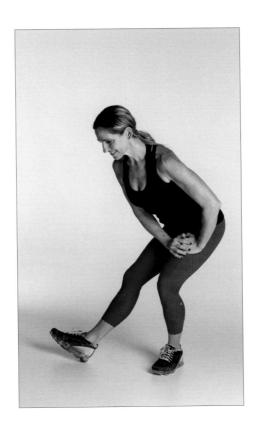

Calf Stretch With Rotation

Benefits

The calf muscles are constantly working. If they tighten, they can restrict motion in both the ankle and hip. The side-to-side movements of this dynamic stretch lengthen the muscles in two planes of motion, sagittal and transverse, to ensure optimal mobility and function of the ankle joint.

Instructions

1. Stand with your feet hip-width apart. Extend your left leg behind you and press your left heel into the ground; place your right leg in front of your body and press your right foot into the ground to enhance stability.
2. Keeping your spine long, use your arms to rotate your shoulders and trunk to the right over your hips; the movement of your torso will help stretch the top of the calf muscles. As you rotate to your right, reach across your body with your left hand (a). Hold the end range of motion for 1 to 2 seconds.
3. Rotate to your left as you reach your right hand to increase the range of motion (b). Hold the end range of motion for 1 to 2 seconds. Perform 8 to 10 repetitions to each side. Switch legs.

Correct Your Form

Make sure the heel of the back foot (the right foot in the instructions) stays on the ground and the back knee stays extended throughout the movement. Move your other leg with a slow, rhythmic motion.

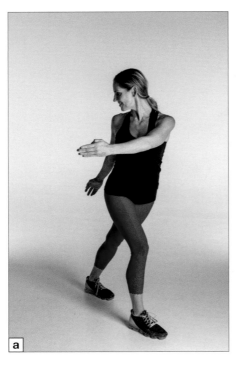
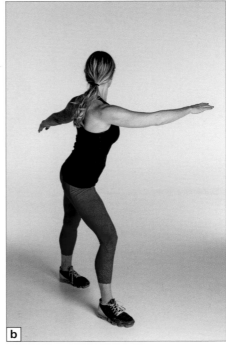

Wide Adductor Stretch

Benefits

The adductors connect from the base of the pelvis to the posterior (back) side of the femur (thigh-bone) and are responsible for both flexing (moving forward) and extending (moving backward) the hip. When the leg is in front of the body, the adductors create hip extension; when the leg is behind the body, the adductors can flex the hip. If the adductors become tight, they can pull the pelvis out of position and change the motion of the hip joint. Lengthening the adductors can improve hip mobility while allowing optimal function of the glutes.

Instructions

1. Stand with your feet parallel and wider than shoulder-width apart, and slide your right foot forward slightly so the heel of the right foot is in line with the toes of the left.
2. Push your left heel into the ground to straighten your left leg while shifting your weight sideways into your right hip.
3. To take the stretch deeper into your left adductors, rotate your shoulders and trunk to your right while pushing the left heel down. Hold the stretch for 30 to 45 seconds; then switch legs.

Correct Your Form

Make sure your feet stay parallel, and keep your left leg straight while pressing your left heel down to increase the stretch response. Rotating to look away from the straight leg (the left leg in the instructions) increases the stretch; maintaining a tall spine will allow you to rotate more easily.

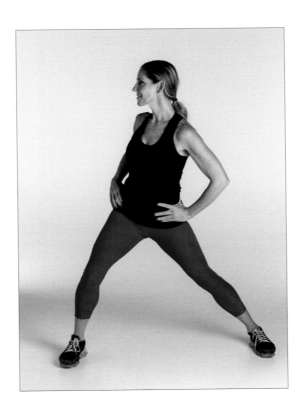

Dynamic Mobility Exercises

According to the law of reciprocal inhibition, the contracting muscles on one side of a joint will inhibit the muscles on the opposite side of the joint, allowing them to lengthen, which can in turn increase joint ROM. Moving joints through their functional ROM can be one of the most effective ways to reduce muscle tightness and improve overall mobility while getting an effective bodyweight strength training workout. The purpose of the following exercises is to improve overall mobility by using movements that involve upper and lower body segments working together. These mobility exercises can be performed as a dynamic warm-up before a high-intensity strength or power training workout or as active recovery the day after a challenging workout. When using them as a dynamic warm-up, complete one to two sets of each exercise; for a stand-alone workout, perform three to four sets of each exercise. Table 4.3 provides a sequence of dynamic mobility exercises to improve overall mobility.

Table 4.3 **Dynamic Mobility Exercise Sequence**

Exercise	Sets	Repetitions
Hurdle walk	2	6-10 steps each direction
Lateral lunge with hip shift	2	6-8 each leg
Forward lunge with reach for ground	2	6-10 each leg
Lateral lunge with same-side trunk rotation	2	6-10 each leg
Transverse lunge with reach for ground	2	6-10 each leg
Reverse crossover lunge with reach for ground	2	6-10 each leg
Hinge to squat	2	6-10

Hurdle Walk

Benefits

Think of hurdle walking as a standing version of supine hip circles (page 68); as you pick up one leg and rotate it at the hip, you press the stance leg into the ground, which helps increase mobility in both hips at the same time.

Instructions

1. Pick up your right foot, and move it forward to create internal rotation of the hip, as if you're stepping over a low fence.
2. As you rotate your right hip, press your left foot firmly into the ground to increase the ROM. If you have room to walk, alternate legs while stepping forward 6 to 10 steps. If room is not available, move the right leg forward and backward before switching legs.
3. Perform the movement backward by pressing the stance leg into the ground as you rotate your upper body to the side of the moving leg; alternate legs as described previously.

Correct Your Form

To achieve the best results, keep your spine tall and long as you walk. As you pick up one leg, squeeze the glutes on the stance leg and move slowly to control your balance.

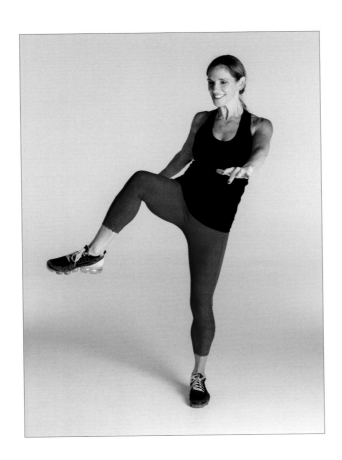

Lateral Lunge With Hip Shift

Benefits

This exercise moves the hips in the frontal plane, helping to lengthen the muscles while improving overall mobility of the joints.

Instructions

1. Stand with your feet hip-width apart, and perform a lateral lunge directly to your left. As your left foot hits the ground, push your left hip back so that your left knee bends as you reach for your left foot with your right hand while straightening your right leg (a).

2. At the bottom of the lunge, push your left foot into the ground to shift your weight to the right into the right hip. Use your left hand to reach for your right foot (b). When your weight is on the right leg, push the right foot into the ground and straighten the right leg as you bring your left foot next to the right to return to standing.

3. Perform a lateral lunge directly to your right and sink into the right hip while reaching for the right foot with your left hand and straightening your left leg. At the bottom of the lunge, push your right foot into the ground to shift your weight to the left into the left hip as you reach for the left foot with your right hand. Push your left foot into the ground to return to standing as you bring your right foot next to your left.

4. This is one rep; perform 6 to 8 reps.

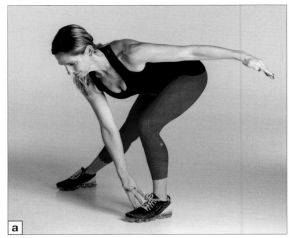

Correct Your Form

The focus of the movement is shifting from one hip to the other at the bottom of the lunge; when shifting from the left to the right, press your right foot into the ground to help pull your pelvis to the right, and vice versa.

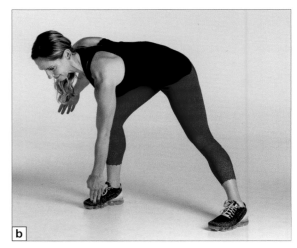

Forward Lunge With Reach for Ground

Benefits

Hinging from the hip while reaching forward and keeping your back heel on the ground will lengthen the hamstring and adductor muscles on the posterior side of your back leg from the calf up to the base of your pelvis. The tension you create as you reach forward to lengthen the muscles in the straight back leg will strengthen the fascia and connective tissues that surround those muscle fibers.

Instructions

1. Stand with your feet hip-width apart, and step forward to lunge with the right leg while keeping your left foot pressed into the ground.
2. As your right foot hits the ground, hinge at the hip and lean forward while reaching as low as possible with both hands (think about trying to reach down to tie the shoe on your right foot while keeping your back leg straight). Keep your left heel pressed into the ground to lengthen the muscles along the back of the left leg.
3. Push off with your right leg and pull yourself back with your left leg as you return your spine to a tall, upright position.
4. Step forward with the left leg while keeping the heel of the right foot flat on the ground. Reach toward the ground in front of your left foot. Perform a total of 6 to 10 reps, then switch legs.

Correct Your Form

Do not let the heel of your back foot come up as you perform this exercise. Keeping your back heel flat on the ground lengthens the muscles of the hamstrings and calves, allowing them to strengthen while stretching. When lunging forward with your front foot, as the foot hits the ground, the initial movement should be the right hip flexing (bending) as your weight sinks back into the right hip before you bend forward. This will reduce strain on the spine.

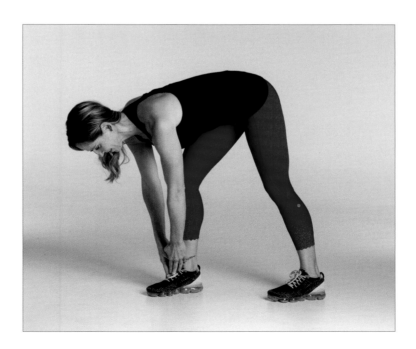

Lateral Lunge With Same-Side Trunk Rotation

Benefits

In this exercise, your shoulders rotate over your hips in order to improve mobility in your hips and thoracic spine at the same time. This exercise can help increase mobility and reduce tightness in your upper back after you have been in a seated position for long periods.

Instructions

1. Stand with your feet hip- to shoulder-width apart. Step directly to your left to perform a lateral lunge, place your left foot on the ground parallel to the right, and let your left knee bend as you sink your weight into your left hip while keeping your right foot pressed into the ground.
2. With your arms in front of your body, rotate your trunk as far as possible to your left while pulling your left arm back to increase the stretch. At the end ROM, pause for a moment before rotating back to face forward.
3. Push off with your left foot as you press your right foot into the floor to pull your body back to the starting position.
4. Perform 6 to 10 repetitions, then switch to the right leg and rotating your trunk to the right.

Correct Your Form

Keep your feet parallel to one another during the lateral lunge: When you lunge to your left, your right foot should point straight ahead, and your left foot should remain parallel to the right foot as it hits the ground. Maintain length through the spine; the straighter the spine, the easier it will be to rotate (rotating while slouching could cause back discomfort). Keep your planted foot pressed into the floor; when lunging to your left, pressing your right foot into the floor will help improve mobility of the right hip.

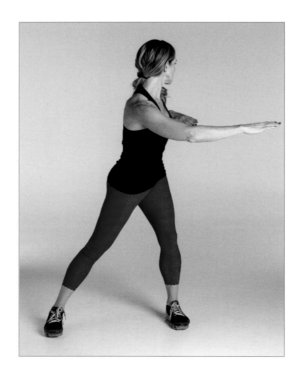

Transverse Lunge With Reach for Ground

Benefits

Rotating from the hips while reaching for the ground can help improve mobility in the hips and upper back at the same time. This move can also strengthen the muscles of the inner and outer thigh in a way that helps to strengthen the fascia while reducing the risk of a strain or an overuse injury to these muscles.

Instructions

1. Stand with your feet hip- to shoulder-width apart (*a*). Lunge your right foot back away from the left foot and place it on the ground pointing toward three o'clock.
2. As your right foot hits the ground and your weight shifts into your right hip, keep your left foot pressed into the ground while squeezing your left thigh to help control stability of the knee.
3. Push your right hip back while you hinge at the hip and lean forward to reach for the ground directly in front of your right foot with your left hand (if you can't reach all the way to the ground, reach for a location in front of your knee; *b*). It doesn't matter whether you actually reach the floor; the important thing is to ensure that the flexion comes from the hip first and the spine second.
4. Return to the starting position by pressing your left (forward) foot down into the ground while squeezing the inner thigh muscles and pushing off with your right foot.
5. Return to the starting position before performing the next lunge. Perform 6 to 10 repetitions on one leg before switching.

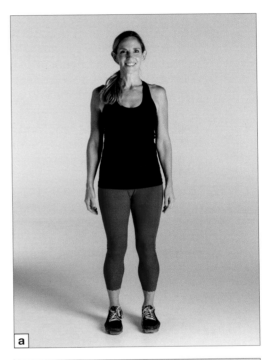

Correct Your Form

Don't allow the front foot to move as you shift your weight onto the foot you are planting; keep the front foot pressed into the ground so it remains pointed forward. Rounding your back to reach for the ground before you create proper hip flexion could cause discomfort in your back; when stepping to your right, make sure that the right hip is flexed and your weight is on your right leg before rounding the spine to reach for the ground.

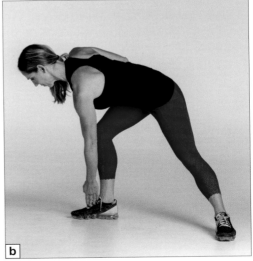

Reverse Crossover Lunge
With Reach for Ground

Benefits

This movement lengthens the muscles of the outer thigh and low back to improve their strength and helps you to control movement at your hips more effectively. Reaching for the ground lengthens the tissues, which can make them stronger and more injury resistant.

Instructions

1. Stand with your feet hip-width apart. Keeping your spine long, move your right foot behind you to the far left side of your left foot (guide your right foot toward seven or eight o'clock), bending your left knee and sinking into your left hip (a).
2. When the ball of your right foot hits the ground, hinge forward at your hips, and reach with the right hand for your left foot (once you have hinged from the hips, you can safely allow your spine to bend; b).
3. To return to standing, press your left foot into the ground as you pick up your right leg and place it back in the starting position. Perform 6 to 10 repetitions stepping with the right leg behind the left before switching to the left leg stepping behind the right.

Correct Your Form

The purpose of this exercise is to use the position and leverage of your mobile leg (the right leg in the instructions) to help increase flexion in your stationary hip (your left hip in the instructions). When sinking into the lunge, push your hips back so that your weight goes backward into your glutes rather than forward onto your left knee.

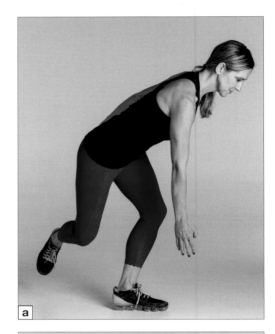

a

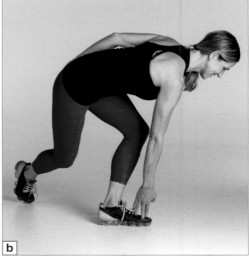

b

Hinge to Squat

Benefits

The hinge and squatting action of this move help to improve hip mobility. Force is transmitted from the ground up through the legs and hips and onto the shoulders and arms. As the hips increase ROM, stronger, more powerful upper body muscles can result.

Instructions

1. Stand with your feet approximately shoulder-width apart, your knees slightly bent, and your hands behind your head with your elbows pointed out to each side.
2. Keeping your spine long, push your hips back to lower yourself into a hinge (your knees should remain slightly bent but not move; *a*).
3. As you hit the end of the hinge, drop both hands to the ground (or as low as possible) before sinking your bottom down into a squat (placing your hands on the ground helps provide feedback for motion from your hips; *b*).
4. From the bottom of the squat, place your hands back behind your head (to stretch the chest) and press both feet into the ground as though you are trying to push the floor away from you. Straighten the legs to return to standing. Perform 6 to 10 repetitions.

Correct Your Form

If lowering yourself into a squat is a challenge, just focus on doing the hinge; hinging from the hips can help improve mobility of the joints while strengthening the large extensor muscles.

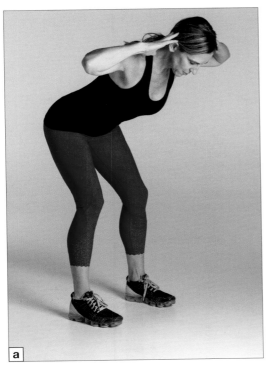
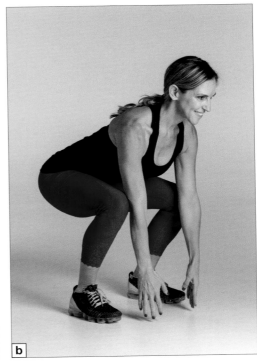

5

Strength and Power Training Methods

How much would you pay for a pill that could greatly reduce the risk of premature death while also slowing down the aging process?

Scientists are working hard to create that pill; however, they can save their time and effort because a solution already exists that may significantly decrease the risk of an early death while changing how the aging process affects the human body. That solution is performing resistance training to enhance strength and power; strength training requires lifting heavy loads to increase the magnitude of muscle force production while power training is the use of explosive movements to accelerate the rate of force development (RFD). Instead of waiting for pharmaceutical companies to invent a pill that *might* slow down the aging process (with numerous side effects, no doubt), you have the ability to slow it down yourself by adding both heavy strength training and explosive, power-based exercises to your current workout routine. According to the 2019 position statement on resistance training for older adults from the National Strength and Conditioning Association (NSCA), the research on exercise for older adults suggests that "countering muscle disuse through resistance training is a powerful intervention to combat the loss of muscle strength and muscle mass, physiological vulnerability and their debilitating consequences on physical functioning, mobility, independence, chronic disease management, psychological well-being, quality of life and healthy life expectancy" (Fragala et al. 2019).

Successful Aging

The concept of successful aging, first proposed by Rowe and Kahn (1998), refers to a reduced risk of disease, ongoing maintenance of physical and cognitive performance, and actively engaging with life. As noted in their research, "To succeed in something requires more than falling into it; it means having desired it, planned it and worked for it. All these factors are critical to our view of aging which, even in this era of human genetics, we regard as largely under the control of individuals" (Rowe and Kahn 1998). Although there will still be some natural muscle loss that comes with age, regular strength workouts can reduce that loss to less than 2 percent per decade (McDonald 2019).

There's even more really good news about strength training. Researchers from the Penn State College of Medicine, Penn State Health Milton S. Hershey Medical Center, and Columbia University who reviewed death data from the 1997-2001 National Health Interview Survey (NHIS) produced by the United States Center for Disease Control found that adults who met twice-weekly strength training guidelines significantly lowered their odds of dying. More than 9 percent of older adults reported strength training at least two times per week during the survey period and, according to the data, those who did had 46 percent lower odds of death for any reason than those who did not participate in strength training. In addition, the adults surveyed who regularly strength trained had 41 percent lower odds of cardiac death and an almost 20 percent reduced risk of dying from cancer. Those in the study group who participated in strength training were also more likely to have normal bodyweight, engage in aerobic exercise, and abstain from alcohol and tobacco (Kraschnewski et al. 2016).

It's time to make a major paradigm shift in how we as a society think about exercise. If you're in your 40s or beyond, forget about the mirror and the scale, and start thinking of every workout as taking a magic pill capable of extending the length and quality of your life. Just as a car that's abandoned will rust and fall apart, a sedentary lifestyle with minimal physical activity can accelerate the aging process and take a devastating toll on your body. There are never any guarantees for how long you will live, but the evidence is overwhelming that a sedentary lifestyle with little to no exercise, poor nutrition, and risky habits like smoking or drinking excessive amounts of alcohol will certainly lead to a premature death (McDonald 2019; Taylor and Johnson 2008).

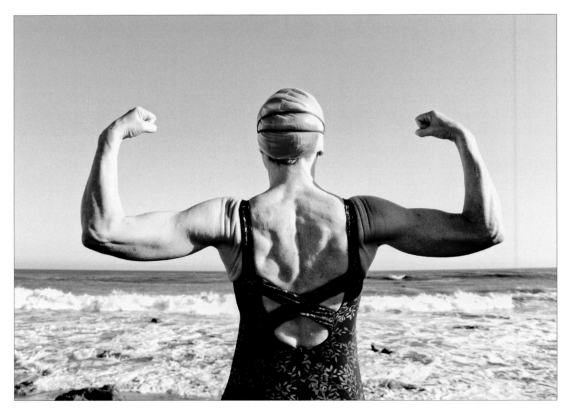

There are no guarantees that exercise will provide specific results, but there is overwhelming evidence that a lack of regular exercise can accelerate the aging process and result in a shorter lifespan.
Peathegee Inc/Tetra images RF/Getty Images

How Resistance Training Changes the Body

One classic 1980s movie that can provide some insight into how resistance training affects the body is *The Terminator*, released in 1984, directed by James Cameron, and starring Arnold Schwarzenegger. Arnold plays the title character: a cybernetic organism (cyborg), a robot designed to look like a human, sent from the future to eliminate a potential adversary. This character, a T-800 model 101 Terminator, is an unfeeling machine controlled by artificial intelligence (AI) that is focused on fulfilling its mission.

In science fiction, a cyborg is controlled by a computer that determines all of the actions the machine performs for its assigned task; in the case of the Terminator, that task is the elimination of Sarah Connor, who is supposed to give birth to a leader of the future rebellion of humans against the machines that rule the earth. The Terminator character in the movie provides a rough analogy for how the natural human body functions.

In the human body, the organs, skeleton, muscles, and fascia are all composed of various types of tissue that can be considered hardware, much like the metal framework of the Terminator character. The central nervous system (CNS), composed of the sensory neurons that receive information and the motor neurons that initiate muscle actions, can be considered the software, or more specifically the operating system that controls the functioning of the hardware (muscles and other tissues). In a computer, operating speed can be improved by installing high-speed processors that take less time to turn sensory input into motor output. In the human body, efficiency of information processing can be improved through exercise, specifically strength and power training.

Strength and power exercises can enhance how your processor (brain) works with the mechanics (muscles and connective tissues) and chemistry (hormones) of your body to promote the growth of new muscle. Resistance training is the application of mechanical forces to the body, which responds by producing more of the chemicals (hormones) that promote the growth of new muscle. Not only can strength and power exercises help improve the speed at which the CNS functions to activate muscles, but as the following paragraphs demonstrate, they could also help stimulate production of new cells so that your body can repair damaged tissues.

The Overload Principle

To achieve the desired results from an exercise program, you need to push your body to work harder than it is used to working. This is known as overload. The overload principle dictates that achieving results from exercise requires gradually increasing the intensity applied to the body so the physiological systems are capable of performing a greater amount of physical work (Haff and Triplett 2016). To increase your muscular strength, you need to exercise with increasingly heavier loads so that you are applying a physical stimulus greater than the neuromuscular system is accustomed to receiving. The physiological response to an overload is muscles becoming able to perform more work.

Research can provide a general guide as to how the body may respond to a specific type of exercise, but the fact is that each of us will experience a slightly different response to strength and power exercises. The ability to increase an individual's level of lean muscle is based on a number of different variables, including gender, age, resistance training experience, genetics, sleep, nutrition, hydration, and other emotional and physical stressors, each of which can change how an individual's physiological systems adapt to resistance training. For example, too much stress at work or a lack of sleep could significantly reduce the ability to grow muscle. Understanding how stress affects muscle growth can help you plan your long-term workout program, discussed at length in chapter 8.

Mechanical stress refers to the physical stresses applied to individual muscle fibers. As depicted in figure 5.1, strength training, specifically the mechanical stresses induced by using external resistance, causes microtrauma to muscle tissue, which in turn signals the biochemical reaction to produce new satellite cells responsible for repairing the structures of the muscle tissue as well as building new muscle proteins (Schoenfeld 2013, 2010). In addition, in his research on cellular adaptations to resistance training, Spangenburg (2009) recognized that "mechanisms activated during mechanical loading of muscle signal changes which create hypertrophy [an increase in muscle fiber size]."

Metabolic stress occurs as the result of a muscle producing and consuming the energy required to fuel contractions. The moderate-intensity, high-volume training programs responsible for muscle growth rely on the glycolytic pathway for energy production. After digestion, carbohydrates are transferred through the blood as glucose and stored in the liver and muscle cells as glycogen. Glycolysis is the process of metabolizing glucose into adenosine triphosphate (ATP), the chemical of energy that fuels muscle contraction, and can occur with oxygen (aerobic) or without (anaerobic). A by-product of anaerobic glycolysis is an accumulation of lactic acid and hydrogen ions, which changes blood acidity, creating acidosis. Evidence suggests a strong relationship between blood acidosis and elevated levels of growth hormone (GH) that support muscle protein synthesis. In their review of the research, Bubbico and Kravitz (2011) noted that "metabolic stress, a result of the byproducts of anaerobic metabolism (i.e., hydrogen ions, lactate and inorganic phosphate) is now also believed to promote hormonal factors leading to muscle hypertrophy."

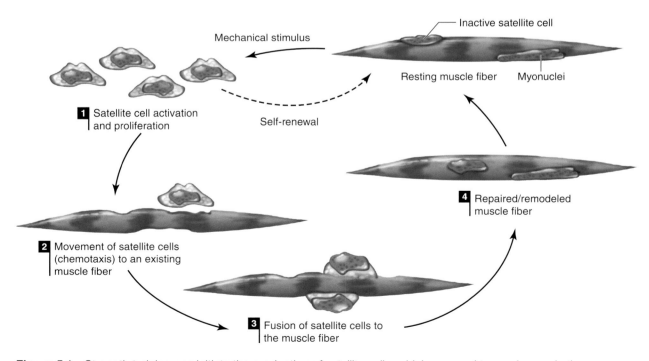

Figure 5.1 Strength training can initiate the production of satellite cells, which are used to repair muscle tissue damaged during resistance training. This repair process can help muscle tissue remain functional well into your later years.

Hypertrophy

Strength and power training create mechanical and metabolic stress, which are two specific types of overload that could result in hypertrophy, an increase in muscle size. There are two specific types of hypertrophy: myofibrillar and sarcoplasmic. Myofibrillar hypertrophy refers to the increase in size or thickness of individual actin and myosin protein filaments, which can improve the force production capacity of the myofibrils. Myofibrillar hypertrophy does not necessarily lead to larger muscles; rather, it results in thicker muscle fibers capable of generating more force. Sarcoplasmic hypertrophy is an increase in the volume of the semifluid interfibrillar substance in the intercellular space that surrounds individual muscle fibers. This fluid contains the proteins used to promote tissue repair and growth. Sarcoplasmic hypertrophy can cause the cross-sectional area of muscle fibers to increase, but most of the enhanced size is due to an increase in volume of the sarcoplasm and noncontractile proteins not directly involved with force production. Resistance training with heavy loads to fatigue can result in a combination of myofibrillar and sarcoplasmic hypertrophy (Schoenfeld 2016; Zatsiorsky, Kraemer, and Fry 2021).

Mechanotransduction is the technical term that describes how mechanical forces create the chemical reactions that lead to muscle growth. In the case of human muscle tissue, forces applied from external resistance damage actin-myosin protein filaments, which in turn initiates the biochemical reactions responsible for repairing the muscle tissue as well as forming new muscle proteins. As researchers have observed, "Mechanical tension may be the most important factor in training-induced muscle hypertrophy. Mechanosensors are sensitive to both the magnitude and duration of loading and these stimuli can directly mediate the intracellular signaling to bring about hypertrophic adaptations" (Schoenfeld 2016).

Strength Training

Strength training is the process of exercising with external resistance for the purpose of enhancing the functional performance of muscle, improving physical appearance, or a combination of the two and is a primary reason why many individuals start a workout program. Strength training can both improve force output (strength) and increase muscle size simultaneously; however, there is a distinct difference between the types of exercises required for each outcome. Strength training with heavy loads can improve muscle force output without necessarily increasing muscle size, while exercising with lighter loads can enhance muscle size without necessarily increasing muscle strength significantly.

Strength training has been used for years as a way to change physical appearance. However, there is strong evidence to suggest that strength training can provide important health benefits as well. All exercise provides general health benefits, but the evidence is beginning to accumulate that higher-intensity strength and power exercises with external resistance may be more effective for reaching the goal of successful aging. For many reasons, those in their later years who could receive the greatest benefits from such exercises often do not perform them.

One outcome of strength training with heavier weights is activating greater numbers of muscle motor neurons and the fibers to which they attach, collectively called the motor unit. Muscle motor units are the basic CNS component responsible for stimulating individual muscle fibers to slide across one another and create muscle shortening. Strength exercises help the CNS become more efficient at transmitting nerve impulses to muscle motor units and increases the number of motor units activated within a muscle.

When it comes to strength training, the 2018 edition of the *Physical Activity Guidelines for Americans* published by the U.S. Department of Health and Human Services suggests the following:

> Adults should also do muscle-strengthening activities of moderate or greater intensity and that involve all major muscle groups on 2 or more days a week, as these activities provide additional health benefits. As part of their weekly physical activity, older adults should do multicomponent physical activity that includes balance training as well as aerobic and muscle-strengthening activities. (U.S. Department of Health and Human Services 2018)

Health Benefits of Resistance Training

While the common perception is that resistance training is for those interested in increasing muscle size or strength, the evidence is strong that resistance training can help achieve optimal health and successful aging. This means that if you exercise consistently and make resistance training a key component of your workouts, you can spend your hard-earned money on things you enjoy as opposed to giving it to pharmaceutical companies for medication to address various health concerns. Remember that the heart is a muscle; just as resistance training strengthens the skeletal muscles that move your body, it can strengthen your heart, improving its ability to move blood around the body and potentially reducing your risk of developing heart disease or other chronic conditions like high blood pressure or high cholesterol. In an extensive review of the literature on the relationship between muscle strength and all-cause mortality, Volaklis, Halle, and Meisinger (2015) documented that multiple study participants who scored higher on strength tests had lower risks of experiencing an early death.

General Health Benefits of Resistance Training (Both Strength and Power)

Improved cardiorespiratory efficiency—delivery of blood to working muscles

Enhanced neural activation of trained muscles

Improved muscle contraction velocities

Stronger connective tissue (tendons, ligaments, and fascia), which can reduce the risk of injury

Improved bone mineral density

Elevated levels of anabolic hormones responsible for muscle growth

Enhanced physical function

Activation of type II muscle fibers, which can atrophy during the aging process

Increased energy expenditure

Muscle hypertrophy and definition

Resistance training could also help to strengthen your brain and reduce the risk of some chronic diseases such as dementia. Lifting weights to the point of fatigue or performing explosive exercises could increase the hormone insulin-like growth factor-1 (IGF-1), which is related to the production of brain-derived neurotrophic factor (BDNF), a protein responsible for stimulating the growth of new neurons in the brain and enhancing communication between existing pathways. In short, lifting heavy could make you smarter by elevating levels of brain-building chemicals. According to a study conducted by Church and colleagues (2016) that looked at how high-intensity and high-volume resistance training affected the BDNF response in the body, "Results indicate that BDNF concentrations are increased after an acute bout of resistance exercise, regardless of training paradigm, and are further increased during a seven week training program in experienced lifters."

Power Training

While lifting weights can increase both, strength and power are two very different outcomes. During a strength exercise, the muscle fibers shorten and lengthen to generate the mechanical forces required to move an external resistance. During a power exercise, the contractile element of muscle tissue (the actin-myosin proteins responsible for contractions) shortens and remains in a shortened position (an isometric contraction), which, in turn, places tension (a lengthening force) on the fascia and elastic connective tissues that surround individual muscle fibers. It's this tension that is actually responsible for generating the forces to create explosive movement. As the fascia and elastic connective tissues are rapidly lengthened, they store mechanical energy, which is then released as the tissues return to their original length. Strength training increases the force produced by the contractile element, helping to enhance the amount of energy that can be stored and released by the elastic tissues. Power exercises can help increase overall force output of muscle tissue and improve the resilience of elastic connective tissues and ligaments, helping to reduce the risk of injuries like muscle strains.

Power training increases the velocity of muscle motor unit activation, thereby improving neural efficiency, or the speed at which the CNS communicates with muscle tissue. Both strength and power training can increase muscle force output; the major difference is that strength training requires the use of heavier weights while power training relies on moving at a faster velocity. Strength training can enhance muscle force production and increase muscle size, helping to minimize the effects of aging-related muscle loss while also improving physical function. However, to enhance your overall ability to perform many activities of daily living (ADLs), it is also necessary to include power training in your exercise program.

How to Increase Strength and Power Output

By improving the coordination and timing of when motor units contract, the CNS is a critical component of increasing both strength and power (figure 5.2). Muscle spindles are sensory receptors that identify changes in muscle length and then communicate those changes to the CNS to determine and produce the appropriate motor response. Muscle spindles lie parallel to individual muscle fibers and sense changes in muscle length as well as the velocity of the length change. When a muscle is lengthened, it stretches the muscle spindles, which respond by initiating a discharge of alpha motor neurons, which in turn cause a reflexive contraction of the involved muscle (Verkhoshansky and Siff 2009). Not only may power training help increase the speed of muscle contraction, but it could also result in muscle growth. In research conducted on the benefits of explosive exercises for older adults, Valls and colleagues (2014) observed that "a resistance training program using moderate to heavy resistance with maximal intentional acceleration of the load (explosive type) is able to improve both strength and power, resulting in higher prescription relevance due to the optimal combination for hypertrophy and neural adaptation effects."

Muscle force output is based not only on the size of the muscle or individual muscle fibers but on *intra*muscular coordination (the efficiency with which the CNS activates individual fibers within a particular muscle), which is based on three separate components:

1. Muscle fiber recruitment: Rapid lengthening during the eccentric phase of the stretch-shorten cycle stimulates muscle spindles to activate higher numbers of muscle motor units within a specific muscle.

2. Synchronization: The activation of greater numbers of motor units simultaneously increases the force output.

3. Rate coding: In general, faster activation of muscle motor units by the CNS leads to an increase in muscle power.

*Inter*muscular coordination is the ability to activate many muscles at the same time in order to achieve maximal force output for a specific movement. CNS adaptations are primarily responsible for increasing both intra- and intermuscular coordination, which ultimately enhances the RFD and total power output for a particular movement. Cocontraction is the simultaneous activation of muscles on both sides of a joint (traditionally referred to as the agonist and the antagonist) for a particular movement. Increasing the neural efficiency of muscles can allow an antagonist to relax at a faster rate during an agonist muscle action, leading to an increased RFD and a faster movement velocity (Verkhoshansky and Siff 2009).

Applying the Terminator analogy, helping a cyborg to increase its strength would require adding more components that can generate force; in the human body, consistent strength training can help enhance the size of muscles and increase the amount

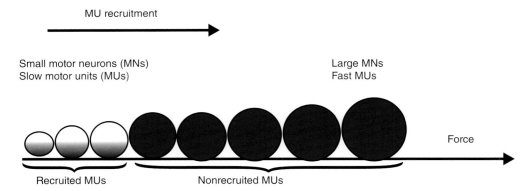

Figure 5.2 Motor neurons (MNs) are the connection between the central nervous system (CNS) and muscular system; they transmit the signal that causes a muscle to contract. A motor unit (MU) is made up of a motor neuron and the muscle fibers to which it is attached. Smaller motor units contain type I muscle fibers (also referred to as slow twitch because they contract at a slower velocity than type II fibers) and the larger motor units are comprised of type II (fast-twitch) muscle fibers. Exercise to the point of fatigue ensures that all available motor units and muscle fibers are recruited and can help ensure optimal strength and power development as well as muscle growth.

Reprinted by permission from V.M. Zatsiorsky, W.J. Kraemer, and A.C. Fry, *Science and Practice of Strength Training*, 3rd ed. (Champaign, IL: Human Kinetics, 2021), 55.

of force they can generate. Increasing a cyborg's power output (the velocity at which it can produce force) would require changing its software; in the human body, explosive exercises can reduce the amount of time it takes for muscles to contract. Changing your body to become stronger and more powerful requires knowing how to engage the components of muscle responsible for producing force.

Muscle Motor Units

A foundational knowledge of muscle fiber physiology can help you understand how important strength and power exercises are to achieving successful aging. An individual motor unit is comprised of a motor neuron, which receives the commands for action from the CNS, and its attached muscle fibers. A motor neuron receives an action signal from the CNS, causing the attached muscle fibers to shorten and contract (figure 5.3). The two basic classifications of muscle fibers are type I (slow twitch) and type II (fast twitch); and because they are attached to specific muscle fibers, motor units can also be classified as fast or slow twitch. Whether slow twitch or fast twitch, motor units are activated according to the all-or-none theory, which postulates that when a motor unit is stimulated to contract it activates all of the attached muscle fibers (Haff and Triplett 2016).

Slow-twitch motor units have a low threshold for activation and low conduction velocities and are also known as aerobic muscle fibers because they are the ones best suited for long-duration activity requiring minimal force output. This is because they contain slow-twitch, type I muscle fibers that rely on aerobic metabolism of free fatty acids for energy. The slow-twitch muscle fibers are recruited first; when they are unable to generate the forces required for a movement, the larger, type II motor units are activated.

Fast-twitch motor units have a higher activation threshold, are capable of conducting signals at higher velocities, and are better suited to power-based exercises. Type IIb fibers use stored adenosine triphosphate (ATP), the chemical that fuels muscle contractions, to generate a high amount of force in a short time without the use of oxygen, making them completely anaerobic. Type IIa muscle fibers rely on glycolysis, the metabolism of glycogen first into glucose, then into ATP, making them more efficient than type I muscle fibers at producing high levels of force in a short period of time. Type IIa fibers metabolize glycogen (the form in which carbohydrates are stored in muscle cells) to produce energy either with oxygen (aerobic) or without (anaerobic).

One of the most important benefits of high-intensity exercise throughout the aging process is improving the ability of type II muscle fibers to metabolize glycogen for fuel. Low-intensity exercise will rely primarily on aerobic metabolism, which can improve fatty acid oxidation but not glycolysis. Additionally, fast-twitch muscle fibers can store glycogen and water, resulting in

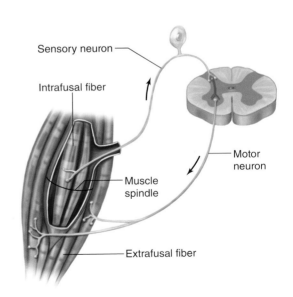

Figure 5.3 One benefit of resistance training throughout the aging process is ensuring optimal communication between the CNS and muscle tissue via the motor neuron.

a greater growth than type I fibers, and are responsible for hypertrophy, the increase in muscle size as the result of strength training. As muscle cells deplete glycogen for fuel during exercise, they will adapt by storing more glycogen during the recovery phase. One gram of glycogen will hold up to three grams of water when stored in muscle cells. Performing repetitions to momentary fatigue, the inability to perform another rep, can deplete stored muscle glycogen, resulting in an increase in muscle size once it is replenished. Recruiting and innervating type II muscle fibers requires creating enough mechanical and metabolic overload to fatigue the involved muscle by the end of the set (Haff and Triplett 2016; Schoenfeld 2016; Zatsiorsky, Kraemer, and Fry 2021).

The initial changes to your body are due primarily to an improved neural function, specifically how many motor units are activated and at what velocity. Strength training increases the number of motor units activated, while power training can speed up their rate of contraction. One of the long-term adaptations of muscle to resistance training is an increase in muscle fiber cross-section. As the cross-sectional areas of type II fibers increase in size from storing more glycogen, they have more surface tension and become capable of generating higher amounts of force.

The Benefits of Unilateral Training

Unilateral refers to using only one arm or leg during an exercise. Performance coaches know the benefits of unilateral exercises for helping athletes improve strength; a technique that could help an athlete earn a scholarship or professional contract is worth considering to achieve successful aging.

It's commonly accepted that unilateral training helps improve strength in the moving limb. Research suggests that the CNS could recruit motor units in the opposite limb at the same time. Studies of this contralateral strength training effect, or cross-education, demonstrate that unilateral strength training could cause a spillover of neural drive to the unused side, resulting in a strength gain (Green and Gabriel 2018; Cirer-Sastre, Beltran-Garrido, and Corbi 2017; Carrol et al. 2006). This means that while you're using your right leg for a split squat or right arm for a one-arm row, the left leg or arm could also be getting stronger even while at rest. Carrol and colleagues (2006) found that "strong contraction of one limb affects the gain of the ipsilateral cortical circuitry that, with repeated execution, could induce adaptations in the 'untrained' control system to allow more effective motor drive when the untrained limb is maximally contracted." Green and Gabriel (2018) observed that "the changes in strength and neuromuscular adaptations were similar between the training and untrained limbs, providing support for the hypothesis that unilateral training induces adaptations of a motor center (such as the premotor cortex) that provides common drive to both hemispheres."

Unilateral exercises could also increase strength of the core muscles responsible for stabilizing the spine and pelvis. When the muscles of a single leg are used to generate the force for an exercise, other muscles are recruited to stabilize the rest of the body while that leg is working. Likewise, when only one arm is used for an exercise, the deep core stabilizers are recruited to create a solid foundation for that arm to move. McGill's research on unilateral movements like suitcase carries, one-arm rows, and one-arm presses suggests that using only one arm for carrying, pulling, or pressing movements could help increase recruitment of spinal stabilizer muscles (McGill 2010; McGill, McDermott, and Fenwick 2009; Santana, Vera-Garcia, and McGill 2007). According to McGill (2010), "While laying, bench press performance was primarily governed by the chest and shoulder musculature, where standing press performance was governed by core strength."

Based in part from P. McCall, *The Benefits of Unilateral Training* (San Diego, CA: ACE).

Classifications of Strength Training

Have you ever noticed that athletes from different strength-based sports have completely different types of muscles? Bodybuilders develop large muscles with impressive levels of definition. Powerlifters generally have large muscles that lack the definition of bodybuilders' muscles, but they are capable of lifting an impressive amount of weight. Olympic weightlifters and track athletes who compete in explosive events can achieve high levels of definition, yet their muscles lack the overall size of bodybuilders' muscles. The differences in body type result from how each individual athlete prepares for competition. Authors Zatsiorsky, Kraemer, and Fry (2021) identify three specific methods of strength training—the maximal effort (ME) method, the dynamic effort (DE) method, and the repeated effort (RE) method—and acknowledge that each can provide different benefits and outcomes for the muscular system. Each type of strength training is summarized in table 5.1, and adding all three to your workout program could help you to age successfully.

Table 5.1 **Classifications of Strength Training Methods**

Method	Description	Intensity	Repetitions
Maximal effort	Using maximum amounts of resistance to create a mechanical overload	85-100% one-repetition maximum (1RM)	1-6
Dynamic effort	Using a nonmaximal load with highest attainable velocity	40-60% 1RM—repeated efforts 80-100% 1RM—single rep efforts	4-8—repeated efforts 1-2—single rep efforts
Repeated effort	Creating a metabolic and mechanical overload by performing repetitions of a nonmaximal load to fatigue	70-80% 1RM	8-12* *Repetitions should be performed until momentary fatigue.

Based on Zatsiorsky, Kraemer, and Fry (2021).

The Maximal Effort Method

The ME method of strength training uses heavy resistance to increase the number of higher-threshold type II motor units activated in a specific muscle. Have you ever felt your muscles shaking as you lifted, or tried to lift, a heavy weight? That happened because the CNS was sending electrical signals to the motor units in an effort to generate the force needed to move the weight. ME training can improve both intramuscular coordination and, when used for multijoint movements like squatting or lunging, intermuscular coordination. The primary stimulus of ME training is mechanical, specifically myofibrillar hypertrophy, which can greatly increase a muscle's force output without adding too much size. Examples of the ME method include the sport of powerlifting, where athletes compete to see who can lift the most weight in three lifts (the barbell deadlift, the barbell bench press, and the barbell squat) and sport strongman (and -woman) competitions, where athletes compete in lifting a variety of heavy things.

The Dynamic Effort Method

The DE method is another way of describing power training; it applies nonmaximal loads moving at the highest attainable velocity to improve overall strength by increasing the RFD from type II muscle motor units. The DE method causes the contractile element of muscle to hold an isometric contraction that places tension on the fascia and elastic connective tissue. The DE method could be the most effective means of increasing the RFD and developing the explosive power that can help you to maintain optimal physical function as you age. In their extensive review of the benefits of resistance training for healthy older adults, Guizelini and colleagues (2018) documented that using a heavier resistance may not be the only method of improving strength and that the velocity of muscle contraction could play an important role in increasing overall muscle force output. Examples of the DE method include Olympic weightlifting, where athletes compete to see who can lift the most weight in the explosive lifts of the barbell snatch and the barbell clean and jerk, and the field sports of shot put, hammer toss, and discus, where athletes compete to see who can throw a weighted implement the farthest.

When muscle cells metabolize fat or carbohydrate into ATP, they are using chemical energy for the contractions; muscles can also produce mechanical energy as a result of the stretch-shorten cycle (SSC) of muscle action. The lengthening (eccentric) phase of the SSC stores potential energy as a muscle lengthens, while the shortening (concentric) phase releases the energy as a muscle returns to resting length. A traditional tempo of exercise is usually one to three seconds each on the eccentric and concentric phases. Power exercises improve the velocity of muscle force production by enhancing the coordination between the contractile and elastic components of muscle, which ends up reducing the time of the SSC. Minimizing the transition time between the lengthening and shortening phases of action increases a muscle's RFD and power output. It is helpful to think of the SSC as a rubber band; a rubber band that is stretched and held in a lengthened position before being released won't produce as much explosive force as one that is rapidly pulled and immediately released.

Additional structural adaptations caused by power training include changes in the quality and quantity of muscle protein and anaerobic enzymes, both of which affect the structure of a muscle. Specific structural changes include increasing the quantity of enzymes necessary for anaerobic metabolism, elevating the amounts of energy substrates such as phosphagen and glycogen stored in muscle, and increasing the contractile proteins of myosin and actin. An additional adaptation is that the myosin heavy chains become thicker, which allows muscle contractions to occur with more velocity and greater amounts of force. Power training not only affects the muscular system but also improves the strength and density of connective tissue such as tendons and ligaments and of the osseous structures of bone (Haff and Triplett 2016).

Using a heavier mass can slow down acceleration but help muscles develop the ability to generate higher levels of force. Using a lighter mass can increase the rate of acceleration, resulting in higher levels of power output.

The Repeated Effort Method

The RE method uses a nonmaximal load lifted repeatedly until the point of momentary muscle fatigue (the inability to perform another repetition). Achieving fatigue helps to ensure that all the involved motor units are recruited. Due to the high rep ranges with a moderately heavy load, the RE method can stimulate muscle growth and strength increases by creating both a mechanical *and* a metabolic overload. In

Newton's Laws of Physics

The different types of resistance training can be explained by applying the basic principles of physics. In general, the faster acceleration of a mass means that a greater amount of force was produced. When muscles accelerate a mass for a specific distance, they are performing physical work. Reducing the amount of time during which work can be performed results in a greater amount of power produced.

1. **Inertia: A body at rest stays at rest unless acted on by an outside force.**

   Applied to exercise, this law explains the fact that a weight will remain at rest until a muscle force is applied to it to produce motion.

2. **Force = mass × acceleration ($F = ma$)**

   Force is the product of a mass and its rate of acceleration; there are two ways to increase muscle force output: Increase the mass by using a heavier load, *or* increase the acceleration by moving the load faster.

3. **Reaction: For every action, there is an equal and opposite reaction.**

   When applied to exercise program design, this law supports the specific adaptations to imposed demands (SAID) principle, which states that the body will adapt (react) to the method in which it is trained (action). For example, athletes who compete in Olympic weightlifting use the DE method to increase their RFD, while powerlifters apply the ME method to increase their overall magnitude of strength.

the RE method, the muscle uses slower motor units for the initial repetitions. As these motor units begin to fatigue, the muscle will recruit higher-threshold type II motor units to sustain the necessary force production. Once the higher-threshold motor units are activated, they fatigue, quickly leading to the end of the set. As anaerobic type IIs are used, they create energy through anaerobic glycolysis, which produces metabolic waste like hydrogen ions and lactic acid, changing blood acidity. Research suggests that acidosis, the change in blood acidity due to an accumulation of blood lactate, is associated with an increase in GH and IGF-1 to promote tissue repair during the recovery phase (Schoenfeld 2013, 2010).

The RE method can produce specific outcomes such as improved energy production and the ability to sustain force over an extended period of time. It's important to note that if the load is not sufficient or the set is not performed to momentary fatigue, then the set will not stimulate the type II motor units or create the requisite metabolic demand promoting muscle growth. Here's good news if you're interested in maintaining or increasing muscle size as you age: In their review of the research literature on the benefits of strength training for older adults, Guizelini and colleagues (2018) found that it is possible for older adults to achieve hypertrophy within three to nine weeks of beginning a resistance training exercise program. An example of the RE method is bodybuilders who perform a high number of repetitions to the point of momentary fatigue in order to increase muscle size and enhance definition.

Based on my observations in commercial fitness facilities, many adults overlook the benefits of all three types of strength training as they age because they have a misconception that the ME and DE methods are only for the young or athletes. Nothing could be farther from the truth! Resistance training for both strength and power could be the key to helping you to achieve successful aging. Going forward, resistance training will refer to both strength and power training, while specific applications for each of the ME, DE, or RE methods will be called out separately.

The ME method can help recruit more motor units and make muscles stronger, the DE method can help increase the RFD and improve explosive power, and the RE method can help add muscle size and change appearance. Therefore, it is important to incorporate all three in your workout programs at various times in order to achieve successful aging; various ways to organize workout programs to include all three will be explored in chapter 8.

It's All Hormones These Days

When you hear the term *anabolic steroids*, you probably think of large, sculpted bodybuilders posing on a stage, gigantic men running into one another on a football field, or overly muscular, costumed performers flying through the air in a professional wrestling ring. Anabolic steroids are perceived as performance-enhancing drugs that athletes take to gain an edge on the competition. However, not only do you have anabolic steroids in your body right now, but you *need* them if your exercise goals include building muscle or increasing your strength.

No, this does not mean that you need to buy products from that shady guy in your gym who seems to be popular with the bodybuilders. Both strength and power training can elevate your natural levels of anabolic (meaning muscle-building) hormones used to repair muscle fibers damaged during exercise. The endocrine system produces the hormones that control cellular function. Mechanical and metabolic stress applied to muscle fibers triggers the endocrine system to increase the production of the hormones responsible for repairing damaged muscle tissue and growing new protein cells. The hormones testosterone (T), GH, and IGF-1 are produced as a response to resistance training because they promote the protein synthesis responsible for repairing and growing new muscle (Schoenfeld 2010; Vingren et al. 2010; Crewther et al. 2006).

Anabolic hormones are those that promote growth (for the record, catabolic hormones are those that break down a substance into smaller components). Steroid hormones interact with receptors in cell nuclei, while peptide hormones work with receptors on cell membranes. Testosterone is an anabolic steroid your body produces that, in addition to other functions, promotes muscle growth by interacting with receptors in the nuclei of muscle cells to help repair muscle proteins damaged during exercise.

Because T promotes sexual development in men, it is classified as an androgen. Testosterone is produced primarily in the Leydig cells of the male testes (hence the name). Women can produce T in the ovaries and adrenal glands but produce much less than men, which means the fear of developing bulky muscles from two or three resistance training workouts per week is unfounded. The technical name for synthetic T taken by those looking to promote rapid muscle growth is exogenous androgen because it is produced outside of the body. Whether you call it an anabolic steroid or an androgen, T is a completely natural substance that enhances muscle growth as part of the normal postexercise repair and recovery process.

There is some good news and some bad news you should know about T, the aging process, and exercise. Let's start with the bad news: As you age, your body will produce less T. Andropause affects men over 30, causing them to produce less T; this explains the seemingly endless number of commercials promoting T-enhancing solutions during televised sports.

Now for the good news: According to research, certain types of exercise can help your body produce T even in your later years. This means that you need to make sure that high-intensity strength training remains a consistent part of your exercise program if you want to maintain T in your body during the aging process. In a study by Baker and colleagues (2006), three age groups of men (20 to 26, 38 to 53, and 59 to 72) performed the same strength training program of six exercises using 80 percent 1RM for three sets of six exercises, 10 reps each. Each group had blood drawn before and after the workout in order to measure how the exercise influenced T production. Prior to the workout, the younger group had a higher level of T, but after the workout, all three groups showed an increase in the hormone, causing the study authors to note, "Middle-aged and older men showed similar relative T responses to those of younger men after a single bout of high-intensity resistance training exercise" (Baker et al. 2006).

Multiple sets of strength training exercises performed to the point of fatigue could be an effective strategy for enhancing T production. According to a literature review by Kraemer and Ratamess (2005), strength training causes the body to make four specific adaptations related to T production: acute changes during and within the first 30 minutes postexercise; long-term changes that increase resting levels of T; long-term changes in how efficiently the body produces T as a result of exercise; and most importantly, an increase in the number of receptor sites that interact with T. As receptor sites increase, there is a better chance for the elevated levels of circulating T postexercise to have an effect on muscle growth. Their research found that a high volume of high-intensity strength training that engages large amounts of muscle mass, combined with relatively short rest intervals of one minute or less, helps to promote T production. The study authors observed that "manipulation of the acute program variables ensures an optimal neuroendocrine response" (Kraemer and Ratamess 2005).

Enhancing the metabolic effect of strength training by reaching the point of fatigue can be an effective way to ensure that the body produces enough T to promote muscle growth. In a separate review of the research literature, Vingren and colleagues (2010) noted that heavy strength training promotes both total T and free T (the levels of the hormone circulating through the bloodstream that can attach to the binding proteins responsible for carrying it to receptor sites in cell nuclei). Supporting the work of Kraemer and Ratamess, they suggested that to promote T, exercise selection should focus on compound movement with shorter rest intervals: "The exercise session should be performed with a heavy resistance hypertrophic-type of loading. Hormonal changes appear to be related to the amount of muscle mass activated and to the metabolic response caused by the exercise" (Vingren et al. 2010).

Stimulus for Muscle Growth

The endocrine system will experience both acute and chronic adaptations to resistance training, both of which are essential for muscle growth. In the acute phase immediately postexercise, the endocrine system will produce T, GH, and IGF-1 to promote repair of the damaged tissue. The long-term endocrine system adaptation is an increase in the receptor sites and binding proteins, which allow T, GH, and IGF-1 to be used effectively for tissue repair and muscle growth (Schoenfeld 2010; Baechle and Earle 2008; Crewther et al. 2006). Researcher Schoenfeld (2010) observed that muscle damage as a result of mechanical tension and metabolic stress from high-intensity exercise is an effective stimulus for producing the hormones responsible for cellular repair and that IGF-1 is "probably" the most important hormone for enhancing muscle growth. Whether the endocrine system is influenced more by mechanical or by metabolic stress is not certain. However, research indicates that organizing the volume and intensity of a training session to feature heavier loads with shorter rest periods can lead to an increase in the production of anabolic hormones promoting muscle growth (Schoenfeld 2013, 2010; Wernbom, Augustsson, and Thomee 2007; Crewther et al. 2006).

There is a scene in *The Terminator* where the cyborg has to repair parts of his body damaged in battle; again, this is where science fiction analogizes a function of the body—in this case, how muscles repair themselves from the damage caused by resistance training. Anabolic hormones play an important role by helping your body produce the fibroblasts (individual cells) used to help to repair existing tissues and build new ones. The rate of this repair and the resultant muscle growth are related to the amount of damage done to the fibers involved in exercise. Moderate to heavy resistance exercises performed at higher repetition ranges can cause more structural damage to the individual actin and myosin protein myofibrils and signal the production of T, GH, and IGF-1 to repair the damage and build new tissue (Crewther et al. 2006).

When we were younger, muscle growth was important for sports or attracting a potential mate. Now that we're aging, we can still pursue muscle growth but for a different purpose: to maintain youthful energy and strength no matter what the calendar says. Yes, the body can experience muscle loss as part of the aging process; however, a growing body of evidence suggests that it is possible to achieve muscle growth in our later years with the use of progressively challenging training loads. The NSCA position statement on resistance training for older adults cites one study where the participants were able to use a full-body strength training program to increase lean muscle mass by an average of 2.3 pounds (1.1 kilograms) of muscle mass per participant during the 20-week study period, even though their average age was approximately 65 (Fragala et al. 2019).

Yes, even in the later years of the human life span, strength training could help your body to become more efficient at producing the hormones that support this process to repair and build muscle (and elevated levels of these hormones can help you to look younger too). Which specific exercises help increase these muscle-building hormones? To achieve successful aging, compound, multijoint strength training exercises like barbell deadlifts, barbell bent-over rows, dumbbell shoulder presses, and kettlebell goblet squats—in addition to explosive movements like kettlebell swings, explosive medicine ball throws, and plyometric jumps—should be the foundation of your workout programs. A number of compound, movement-based exercises and complete workout programs are presented in the next chapter.

6

Strength and Power Exercises and Workouts

When it comes to strength and power training, gravity is an essential component. Gravity, of course, is the ever-present downward force that accelerates us into the earth at about 32 feet per second squared (10 meters per second squared [m/s²]), keeping us from flying off the planet into space. Gravity is also responsible for applying forces to muscles when using exercise equipment. When they contract, muscles generate the force to create movement by accelerating weight against the downward force of gravity.

Barbells (figure 6.1), dumbbells, kettlebells (figure 6.2), medicine balls, cable machines (figure 6.3), rubber resistance, jump boxes, suspension trainers (figure 6.4), sandbags, and weight sleds can all help improve muscle strength and power. One of the toughest challenges in designing an exercise program is knowing which equipment to use and how to use it in order to get the results you want in the safest, most effective way possible. Multijoint, multimuscle movement patterns with free weights like barbells, dumbbells, and kettlebells involve a number of different muscles and can generate both metabolic and mechanical overloads.

From weight plates to an exercise-based virtual reality experience, exercise equipment is nothing more than tools designed for a specific purpose. Almost any piece of exercise equipment can produce benefits when used properly; however, if used carelessly or without the proper technique, that same equipment could easily cause an injury or, in the worst-case scenario, a fatality. Every single piece of exercise equipment has a specific purpose; some equipment is designed to build strength, while other equipment may be better suited for metabolic conditioning or mobility training.

When introducing power training exercises, it can be extremely important to start with a limited volume of low-intensity exercises to allow the musculoskeletal system to adapt to the faster stretch-shorten cycle velocities. Progressing to higher-intensity exercises can yield greater results but require longer rest periods between sets to allow the structural and neural properties of muscle to experience an appropriate recovery.

Power training exercises require the technical skills to rapidly accelerate a mass, and proper technique is critical for achieving optimal benefits with minimal risk of injury. Learning and refining the technical skills required to perform explosive movements can be a lengthy process. Efficient, skilled movement improves technique, which can lead to the ability to achieve greater results by training with heavier loads. Power training exercises include plyometric jumps to develop lower body power, medicine ball throws to improve upper body power, and the snatch and the clean and jerk to enhance total body power output.

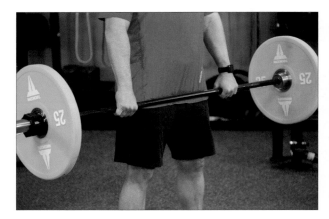

Figure 6.1 Barbell.

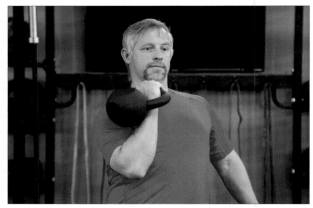

Figure 6.2 Kettlebell.

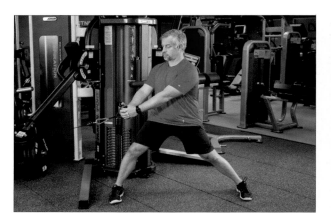

Figure 6.3 Cable machine.

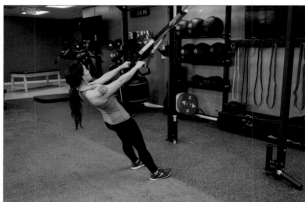

Figure 6.4 Suspension trainer.

Benefits of Strongman Training for Successful Aging

Strength competitions have been around as long as humans have been lifting heavy things. Powerlifting, Olympic weightlifting, and strongman competitions are similar in that they measure an individual's strength and ability to apply muscular force to overcome an external resistance. While weightlifting and powerlifting use a barbell to perform curvilinear movements occurring primarily in the sagittal plane, strongman competitions test an individual's ability to move a number of irregular objects in a variety of different patterns.

Strongman lifting techniques are an example of the relationship between force production and movement skill. Powerlifting and Olympic weightlifting competitions have athletes compete against one another to move a weight in a single plane of motion opposite to gravity; however, in strongman competitions, many of the events require the athletes to move a weight in multiple planes through gravity. While strongman competitions have been held for decades, research suggests that strongman-style exercises may be beneficial for the average fitness enthusiast (Winwood, Keogh, and Harris 2011; Zemke and Wright 2011; Keogh et al. 2010b; McGill, McDermott, and Fenwick 2009). The studies demonstrate the efficacy of strongman-type exercises and provide the rationale for adding them to your workout programs.

Some strongman lifts require strength endurance to maintain force output for a number of repetitions, while others require the generation of a large amount of force in the shortest time possible. For example, a log lift requires competitors to perform an overhead lift for the highest number of repetitions, while Atlas stones competitions require athletes to explosively lift a heavy load to an elevated platform (McGill, McDermott, and Fenwick 2009).

There are a number of different events in a single competition, so strongman athletes need to incorporate diverse strength and power exercises into their contest preparation. Because of their comprehensive approach to training, strongman competitors are able to generate and sustain tremendous amounts of muscle force, and elite-level strongman athletes can be considered among the fittest athletes. In fact, a number of collegiate and professional strength coaches responsible for training athletes incorporate strongman training techniques into their conditioning programs (Winwood, Keogh, and Harris 2011; Zemke and Wright 2011; McGill, McDermott, and Fenwick 2009).

With the exception of the bench press, the lifts used in powerlifting and weightlifting competitions (specifically the squat, the deadlift, the snatch, and the first and second pull phases of the clean and jerk) require a participant to move the weight with his or her feet relatively parallel and approximately hip- to shoulder-width apart. This balanced stance may be an effective way to generate force at the hips for the specific exercises in these competitions; however, many activities of daily living (ADLs) and athletic movements require an individual to apply muscle force with the feet in a variety of positions, very rarely in parallel. Powerlifting and weightlifting emphasize the basic movements of pulling, pushing, and squatting; strongman competitions feature these movements as well as others such as lifting, towing, throwing, swinging a hammer, and walking while carrying heavy objects. Using strongman-type lifts may provide significant benefits by training individuals how to create and use strength in a number of different situations (Zemke and Wright 2011; McGill 2010; McGill, McDermott, and Fenwick 2009).

Research by Keogh and colleagues (2010a) has found that heavy sled pulling can help athletes and sprinters improve acceleration and running speed. Pulling a heavy sled (or vehicle) trains athletes how to maintain a forward-leaning body position while producing the strength to push into the ground one leg at a time and create the horizontal forces necessary to move the sled. This helps explain why many commercial fitness facilities have added space in their workout areas for movements like tire flips, sled pushes, and kettlebell carries and why manufacturers like StairMaster have created products like the HIITMill X that allow users to replicate sled pushes and farmer's carries without the need for an excessive amount of space.

Strength and Power Exercises Based on the Foundational Movement Patterns

This section will provide an overview of strength and power exercises using a variety of equipment such as bodyweight, medicine balls, kettlebells, and cable-based strength training machines. Examples are provided at the end of this chapter of how to organize these exercises into workout programs to achieve successful aging. The exercises are based on the foundational patterns of human movement and, because they incorporate multiple joints and muscle groups, should be the foundation of any resistance training program. These exercises can help develop integrated strength, the ability of multiple muscle groups to work together to generate high levels of force. In addition, using multiple muscle groups at the same time can help increase overall caloric burn, so you will be applying mechanical overload while being more efficient at burning calories.

Hinges and Squats

Hinges and squats are both foundational patterns of movement, and being able to perform a good hinge is essential for being able to squat. When you do a squat, your hips should move back behind your body as your knees move forward; ideally, your spine and shins should be relatively parallel during the movement. If squatting is not comfortable because of previous knee injuries, hinge exercises like the hip thrust and the Romanian deadlift (RDL) can help develop strong hips while reducing vertical compression on the knees.

Barbell Hip Thrust

Benefits

The hip thrust places the greatest amount of force on the glute muscles when the hips are fully extended and those muscles are completely contracted. This exercise is a great option if you experience any low back or knee soreness because those joints do not undergo any vertical compression during the movement the way they do with a squat, lunge, or deadlift.

Instructions

1. Lie faceup (supine) on the floor, and roll the barbell to directly over your hips (it is recommended to use a pad to reduce the pressure of the bar on the pelvis). When the bar is in place, bend your knees toward the ceiling and pull your toes up toward your shins.
2. Hold the bar on your hips as you press your heels down into the ground while pushing your hips up toward the ceiling (a); pause for 2 to 3 seconds at the top before slowly lowering back down to the floor.

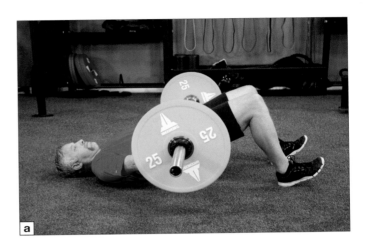

Correct Your Form

If you feel excessive tightness in the back of your legs (the hamstring muscles), move your feet a little farther away from your glutes. Keep both shoulders on the floor during the movement, with your head resting comfortably.

Dumbbells Variation

When using dumbbells instead of a barbell, place them right on top of your hip joints and hold them in place with your hands throughout the entire range of motion (ROM) of the exercise (b).

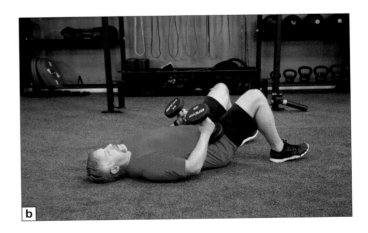

Romanian Deadlift (RDL) With Dumbbells

Benefits

This move strengthens the muscles along the posterior (back) side of the body that help with locomotion and maintaining an optimal posture.

Instructions

1. Stand with your feet hip-width apart, knees slightly bent, and spine straight while holding one dumbbell in each hand so that your hands are resting along the front of your thighs.
2. Keeping your spine long, push your hips back while hinging forward at the hips. Lower yourself until you feel tension in the back of your thighs *or* you feel that your back will start to round (*a*). Your spine should stay straight with your knees bent during the entire movement.
3. To return to the standing position, press your feet into the ground as you push both hips forward.

Correct Your Form

You should feel the work in your glutes as well as in the hamstring and adductor muscles along the back of your thighs. To help maintain a straight spine, think about pulling both shoulder blades down to your tailbone as you hinge forward at the hips. Keep your spine long during the entire movement. Lower yourself until you cannot keep your spine straight; do not allow your spine to bend or round.

Barbell Variation

When using a barbell, grip the bar, with both palms down (pronated), as tightly as possible during the full movement. Start with the bar in front of the thighs, and follow the dumbbell instructions (*b*).

Kettlebell Variation

When using a single kettlebell, grip the handle in a palms-down (pronated) grip. Keep the thumbs next to one another and squeeze the handle as tight as possible during the movement (*c*).

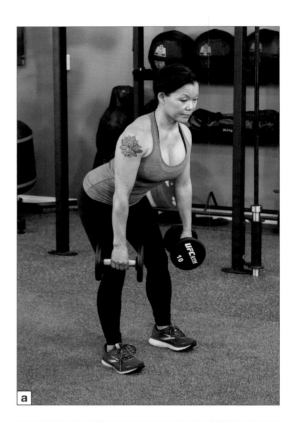

a

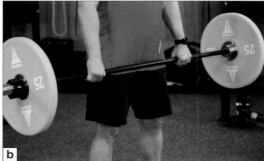

b

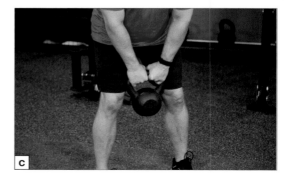

c

Barbell Deadlift

Benefits

The deadlift is so called because the weight is sitting in a "dead," nonmoving position at the beginning of the lift. Because it engages the large muscles of the glutes and upper legs while the spine remains in a stable, nonmoving position throughout the entire ROM, the deadlift is one of the most effective exercises for strengthening the muscles that stabilize and move the core. A deadlift is different from a squat in that the movement primarily involves the hips, with most of the force coming from the glutes; in a squat, the hips and knees move together.

Instructions

1. Stand behind the barbell with your feet approximately hip-width apart and shins touching the bar; grip the bar tightly with both hands in a palms-down (pronated) grip (*a*). Throughout the lift, grip the bar tightly as if you are trying to bend it.
2. Keep your shins vertical and spine long as you sink back into your hips. Gripping onto the bar tightly will help you maintain your balance; if you let go, you may fall back on your tailbone.
3. To lift the bar, press your feet into the ground as though you are pushing the floor away from you while you pull your knees back (to engage your hamstrings) and drive your hips forward. The bar should travel upward in a straight path along the front of your legs (*b*).
4. Stand up until your hips are fully extended. To return to the floor, keep your spine long as you push your glutes back behind you. As you sink back into your hips, keep the bar close to the front of your legs, with your shins vertical.

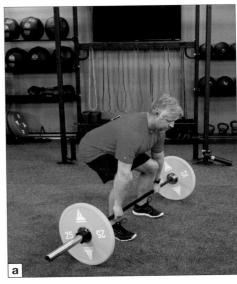

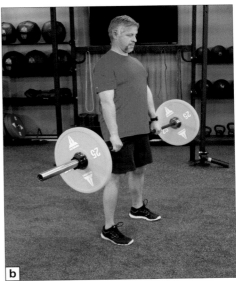

Correct Your Form

As you do the lift, keep your chest lifted and spine long so that you feel the work in your glutes and along the back of your legs. To strengthen your core muscles, use a lighter weight so that you do not have to wear a lifting belt; that way, the deep core muscles, not the belt, are creating the stability for the spine. However, a belt is advised for additional stability when doing maximal loads for three or fewer reps.

Kettlebell Variation

A heavy kettlebell is a great option for the deadlift because the weight will be directly under your center of mass. Grip the top of the kettlebell handle with both hands palms down (pronated) so that your thumbs are right next to each other (*c*). Follow the instructions for the barbell deadlift. The goal is to keep the shins vertical and use your hips to lift the weight.

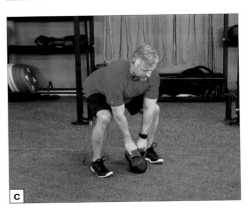

Kettlebell Goblet Squat

Benefits

Holding the weight in front of your body rather than on your shoulders, like for a traditional barbell back squat, is safer for the cervical spine, allows you to keep a better posture during the movement, and helps recruit more of the deep muscles that stabilize your spine, making it a more effective exercise for strengthening your core muscles. In addition, holding a kettlebell (or dumbbell) is more comfortable than a barbell resting on your spine.

Instructions

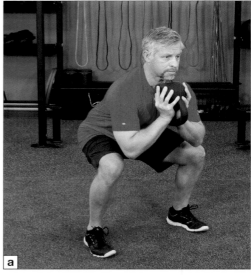

1. Hold a kettlebell in a bottom-up (inverted) position so that the handle is between your forearms. Press your hands into the sides of the bell throughout the lift; this will help to activate your core muscles.
2. Keeping your spine long and chest lifted, sink back into your hips. For stability and to completely engage the deep stabilizers of your core, press your feet into the ground.
3. Allowing your knees and hips to bend simultaneously, lower yourself to a comfortable depth (*a*). To return to standing, straighten your legs and press the floor away from you with your feet.

Correct Your Form

When doing a goblet squat for the first time, use a lighter weight to become comfortable with the weight placement. As you sink into your hips, allow your knees to move forward slightly; the goal should be for your shins and spine to be relatively parallel during the lowering phase of the movement. If you need to, slide a small (5-pound [2 kg]) weight plate under each heel to help make the lift more comfortable for your calves and allow you to have a greater ROM from your hips.

Dumbbell Variation

Hold the dumbbell in a vertical position, keeping your upper arms and elbows close to your rib cage (*b*). Follow the instructions for the kettlebell goblet squat.

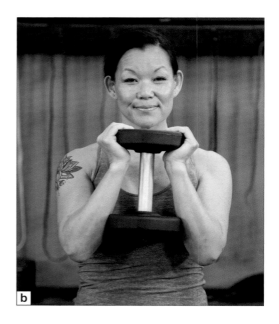

Kettlebell Swing

Benefits

The kettlebell swing is an explosive movement that engages the larger muscles of the lower body, specifically the glutes, hamstrings, adductors, and quadriceps. Because so many muscles are involved in the rapid force production, this exercise can burn a lot of calories. In addition, it's a great exercise for elevating the heart rate and increasing metabolic overload to help promote an increase in the anabolic hormones responsible for muscle growth.

Instructions

1. Place the kettlebell on the ground in front of your body. Grip the handle in both hands, keeping your arms mostly straight with a slight bend in the elbows. Stand with your feet hip-width apart, keeping your knees slightly bent. Squeeze the handle in both hands for a tight grip. Keeping your spine long, hinge your hips to pull the kettlebell back between your legs under your hips, as though you are hiking a football (*a*).
2. Quickly push your hips forward to generate the forward energy to cause the kettlebell to swing up in front of your body (*b*). The strength to move the weight should come from your legs and hips, *not* your shoulders.
3. Allow the kettlebell to come up to chest height before pulling it back down between your legs to prepare for the next repetition. The goal is to move as explosively as possible from the hips.

Correct Your Form

Pulling the kettlebell down quickly can lead to greater activation of your glutes so that you have more power as your hips extend to swing the kettlebell back up; the faster you pull it down, the more explosive your hip extension to lift the kettlebell up toward chest height. Keep your spine long and shins vertical as you move from your hips. If the kettlebell is coming higher than your shoulders, use a heavier weight; using a heavier kettlebell can actually reinforce better form because you cannot cheat the movement.

   Avoid taking the kettlebell all the way to an overhead position into what is typically called the American swing. Moving the arms to an overhead position while holding the weight could actually create impingement of the glenohumeral joints of the shoulders and put you at risk of injury.

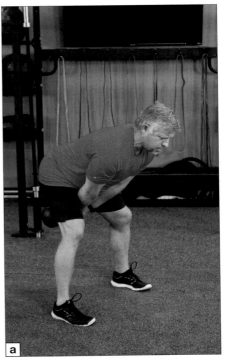
a

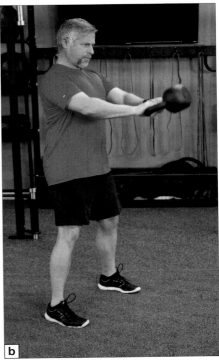
b

Squat Jump

Benefits

This explosive movement engages the type II muscle fibers responsible for rapid force production. The type II fibers metabolize glycogen for fuel, helping your body to become more efficient at using carbohydrates, which can reduce your risk of type 2 diabetes. In addition, explosive jumps can help with dynamic balance to increase overall coordination and body control. One important benefit of using a box is that it can be easier on the body because you are not landing from the height of the jump.

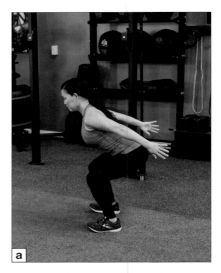

Instructions

1. Stand with your feet hip-width apart. Keeping your spine straight, quickly sink back into your hips while swinging your arms behind your body (a).
2. Explosively swing your arms forward as you press your feet into the ground and snap your hips upward to generate the energy to jump. The energy to jump up should be a combination of your arms swinging forward and your hips rapidly extending as you push the floor away from you (b).
3. To land, let the balls of your feet hit the ground first and then roll down into your heels before sinking back into your hips.

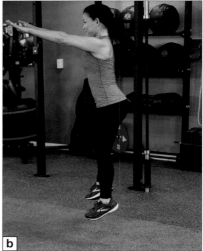

Correct Your Form

To practice proper form, do squats to toe raises: Sink into your hips with your hands behind your body, and slowly stand up as you swing your arms forward. As you reach the standing position, roll up onto your toes (like doing a calf raise); then slowly roll your feet down and lower your arms as you sink back into your hips. Practice 5 to 6 reps before doing the jumps.

Explosive movements are important for activating the type II fibers; the goal is to move explosively, not to jump high. When doing jumps repetitively, let the foot roll all the way down to the heel but minimize your time on the ground. Imagine you're on hot asphalt in the summer: As soon as your foot is all the way flat, explode into the next jump.

Box Jump Variation

Having a target to jump to can help improve overall explosiveness and jump height (c). Start with a box that is lower than knee height. Always jump up and step down from a box; jumping backward is unnecessary. If you are jumping down backward and lose your balance, you have a high risk of falling right back on your tailbone with your heading hitting the ground. It is much safer to focus on the upward explosion of the jump and step down to control your return to the start.

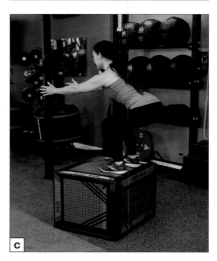

Single-Leg Exercises

The human body functions using only one arm or leg at a time. Gait, the process of walking or running, could be considered the default pattern of human movement; during gait, the body rapidly transitions from one leg to the next. When walking, the only time both feet are in contact with the ground at the same time is during the phase of front-foot heel strike and early back-foot heel off; when running, only one leg makes contact with the ground at a time. Walking (and running) occurs as a result of transitioning the body's weight from one leg to the other. When the muscles of a single leg are used to generate the force for an exercise, other muscles are recruited to stabilize the rest of the body while that leg is working.

Single-Leg Romanian Deadlift (RDL) With Kettlebell

Benefits

Exercising on one leg can improve balance and coordination while engaging the deep core muscles responsible for stabilizing the spine. This move engages the muscles of the inner and outer thigh at the same time, making it time efficient for both strength training and calorie burning. In addition, hinging at the hip while pressing one foot down into the ground can create a deep stretch of the hamstring and adductor muscles along the back of that thigh.

Instructions

1. Stand with your feet hip-width apart, knees slightly bent, and spine fully lengthened. Hold the kettlebell in your left hand, directly in front of your hips.
2. Push your hips backward as you extend your left leg behind you, balancing on your right leg. Keeping your spine long, extend your left foot directly behind you while straightening your left leg.
3. Continue hinging forward from your hips to a comfortable position. Allow the kettlebell to lower to the floor in a straight line directly in front of where your left leg should be.
4. To return to standing, press your right foot into the floor while pulling the bottom of the right side of your pelvis down toward the back of your right leg and returning the left leg to the starting position.

Correct Your Form

Control the forward hinging motion by straightening your left leg, contracting your left thigh, and extending your left foot. Straightening your left leg will help you control the hinge on your right. Keep your spine long throughout the movement.

Dumbbell Variation

The only difference in using a dumbbell is that the handle is the center of mass; squeeze the handle tight to help engage the core muscles and develop greater grip strength.

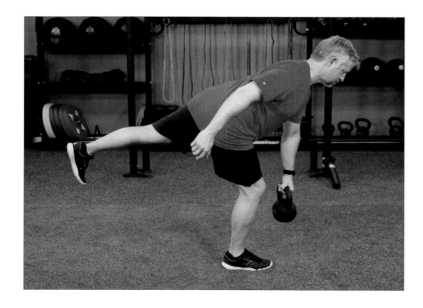

Reverse Lunge With Dumbbells

Benefits

Stepping backward into a lunge creates hip flexion. This recruits more of the glutes, making it safer than traditional forward lunges, which can place more stress on the knee. In addition, the reverse lunge can help to strengthen the hamstring and adductor muscles, creating more stability at the knee joint.

Instructions

1. Stand with your feet hip-width apart and hands by your sides, each holding one dumbbell (*a*).
2. Press your right foot into the ground as you step backward with the left foot, placing the toes of the left foot on the ground.
3. Keeping your spine long, lower your left knee toward the ground (do not let it hit the ground) and sink into your right hip. While lowering, lean forward slightly to increase the amount of work for your glutes (*b*).
4. To return to standing, press your right foot into the ground to pull yourself back up while swinging your left leg forward. Perform all reps on one leg before switching legs.

Correct Your Form

Keep your spine long and straight during the lunge. When returning to standing from the bottom of the lunge, press your standing foot into the ground to pull yourself forward using the muscles along the back of your leg.

Kettlebell Goblet Variation

Hold the kettlebell in both hands in a bottom-up (inverted) position with the handle between your forearms (see kettlebell goblet squat on page 114) and follow the dumbbell instructions. Holding the weight in front of your body can help recruit more of the deep muscles responsible for stabilizing your spine.

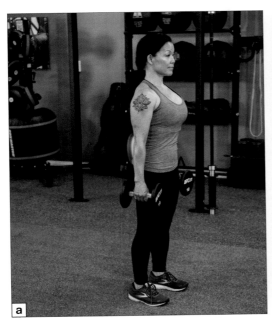
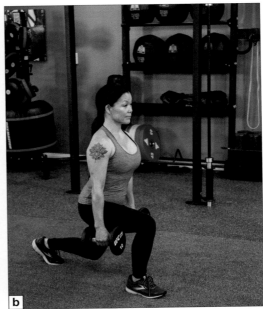

Rear-Foot Elevated Split Squat
With Dumbbells

Benefits

This exercise focuses all of your energy into one leg at a time, which could result in stronger muscles and better coordination. Since you walk and run on one leg at a time, this move helps strengthen your muscles based on how they are designed to function.

Instructions

1. Place the top of your left foot on a box or bench (pictured) positioned behind you at approximately knee height, and press your right foot firmly into the ground. The right foot should be far enough forward that the knee is directly over the ankle joint.
2. Hold one dumbbell in each hand, and keep your spine long as you sink back into your right hip to lower your left knee toward the ground. Your weight should shift back toward the box or bench so that you feel most of the work in your right hip (a). The right knee should bend, but only after the movement has started with the hip.
3. Keep your pelvis level (pressing your foot into the ground helps to recruit the core muscles to control your pelvis) as you lower yourself to a comfortable depth.
4. To return to standing, press your right foot into the ground as you pull your right knee backward (toward the box or bench) to help engage the extensor muscles along the back of the thigh. Perform all reps on one leg before switching legs.

Correct Your Form

Using a box or bench that is too low or too high is a common mistake. Select a box or bench that is at least knee height but no taller than midthigh. To make this a more effective exercise for strengthening your glutes, focus on your weight moving backward toward the box or bench as opposed to forward into the knee joint. The knee of your back leg should be almost directly under the hip while lowering to the ground.

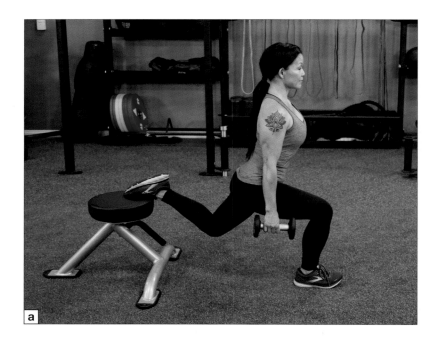

Kettlebell Variation

To increase the level of difficulty and make this a more effective exercise for strengthening your core muscles, hold a kettlebell in the left hand (according to the instructions; as a general rule, hold the kettlebell on the side of your body with the foot on top of the box for best results). Grip the kettlebell tightly to help recruit more core muscles for stability.

Suspension Trainer Variation

Using a suspension trainer can allow you to move your leg farther behind your body, resulting in a greater ROM. Place your left foot in the cradle (the fabric loop of the suspension trainer), and keep your right foot pressed into the ground to engage your core muscles. Press the top of your left foot into the cradle and straighten your left leg behind you to create more stability while lowering yourself into your right hip (b). Pull your left leg forward when returning to the standing position.

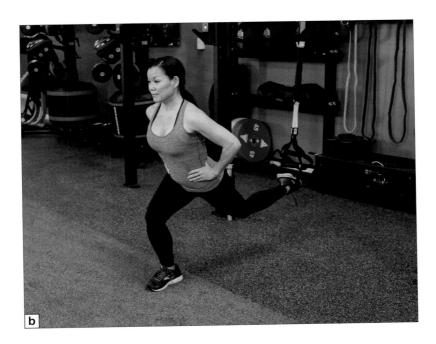

Lunge Jump

Benefits

Lunge jumps use both legs at the same time to develop lower body power. In addition, the cycling action of the movement can help improve overall coordination and movement skill.

Instructions

1. Start in a static lunge position with your right foot forward and your left leg behind your body. Position your left arm forward and right arm back so that they move in opposition to the legs, like when you walk (*a*).
2. Lean forward slightly to lengthen the glutes, and focus on keeping a straight spine throughout the movement. Explosively press your right leg into the ground while driving your right arm forward and left arm backward to create the upward movement.
3. Quickly bring your left leg forward as you move your right leg back so that you land with your left foot in front of your body and your right leg behind (*b*).

Correct Your Form

When learning this exercise, focus on moving your legs quickly as opposed to jumping high in the air; as your skill improves, you can start jumping for height. When landing, let your weight sink back into your hips so that it doesn't go forward into the knees.

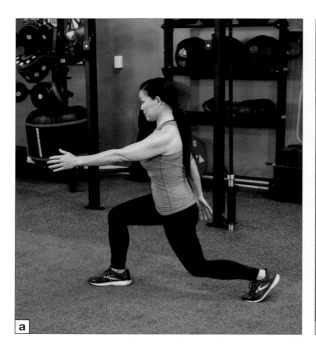
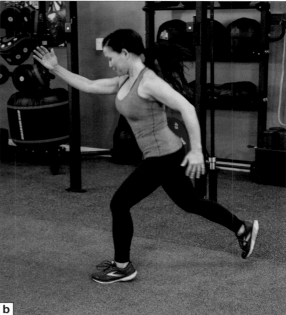

Lateral Bounds (Ice Skaters)

Benefits

When done properly, lateral bounds can help strengthen the outer thigh and lateral hip muscles while increasing your overall energy expenditure. Strengthening the lateral hip muscles can help enhance hip stability for a more powerful running stride.

Instructions

1. Stand with your feet hip-width apart. Keeping your spine long as you sink into a partial squat, pick your left foot off the floor. Explosively push into your right foot (*a*), and then quickly move to your left.
2. Let your left foot hit the ground with the ball of the foot first before rolling down to the heel. As you sink into your left hip, allow your right arm to reach across your body to create more rotation at the hip for stability (*b*).
3. Quickly pull your right arm back to your right side as you explosively push into your left foot and return to the right.

Correct Your Form

When landing from any jump, the sequence should be ball of foot, heel of foot, hip moves backward. As you learn this exercise, start with small movements at a steady pace. You can increase the ROM and pace as the movement becomes more natural. Allow your weight to sink back into your hip when landing rather than letting it move forward into your knee.

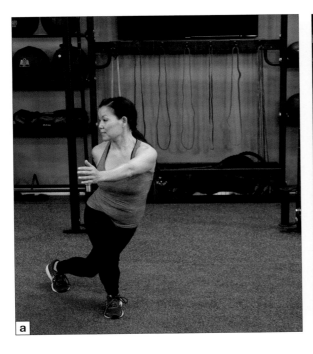

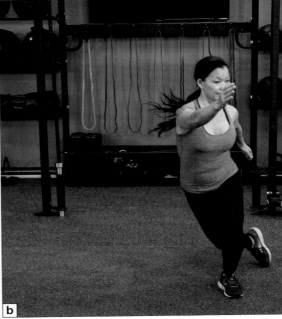

Push Movements

The push movement can take place in two directions: forward and away from the body, like the chest press or push-up, or overhead in an upward direction, like the overhead press. When the feet are firmly planted on the ground in a standing position, as in a standing overhead press, the deep muscles that stabilize the spine will be recruited to create more overall strength. When the hands are on an unstable object like the handles of a suspension trainer, more core muscles will be recruited for stability. Using a bench for traditional chest press movements can restrict the motion of the scapulae (shoulder blades) around the dorsal rib cage, which could cause impingement injuries. If you have any shoulder soreness or a history of shoulder injuries, push-ups may be a better option than a chest press to allow a greater ROM and engage and strengthen all of the muscles responsible for controlling the motion of the joint. As you age, unless you're a competitive powerlifter and how much weight you bench is important, your strength training program should focus more on maintaining optimal shoulder function.

Push-Up

Benefits

The push-up is a foundational exercise that can strengthen the chest, shoulders, and arms while also engaging the deep core muscles responsible for stabilizing the spine. Plus, the push-up can be done anywhere with no equipment, so there is no excuse for skipping a workout. Doing a little bit of something, like a couple of sets of push-ups, is much better than doing a whole lot of nothing.

Instructions

1. Start in the high plank position, legs hip-width apart. Press your hands into the ground with your fingers pointed away from your feet, and contract your thigh and glute muscles to increase stability.
2. Slowly lower yourself toward the floor. Pause at the bottom of the movement (*a*) before pressing your hands into the ground to return to the starting position.

Correct Your Form

Pressing your hands into the ground while contracting your glute muscles can engage the deep core muscles to enhance overall stability. If a full push-up is too challenging, lower yourself with your legs straight, then lower your knees to the ground to shorten the distance between your hands and distal contact point before pushing back up to the starting position.

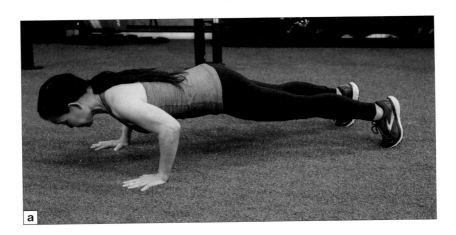

Suspension Trainer Variation

Due to the instability created by a suspension trainer, it is an effective piece of equipment for strengthening the deep core muscles. There are two different ways of doing a push-up with a suspension trainer. The first is by holding on to the handles and placing your feet on the floor (*b*). In this position, the closer to the floor and more horizontal your body, the more resistance you use (the more vertical your body, the less resistance). The key is to squeeze your glute and thigh muscles to create more stability while your toes are the pivot point on the floor.

The second position, placing your hands on the floor and feet in the foot cradles (the fabric loops by the handles), creates a different challenge: You will have more stability in your shoulders while your core muscles will work harder to reduce unwanted movement from your body. Pressing your hands into the floor while pushing your back up toward the ceiling can increase engagement of the core muscles (*c*).

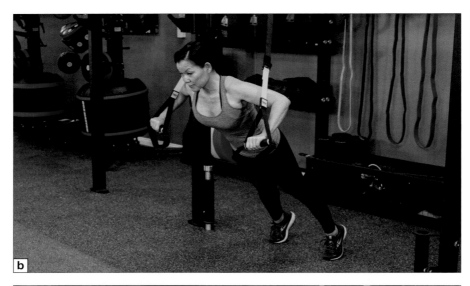

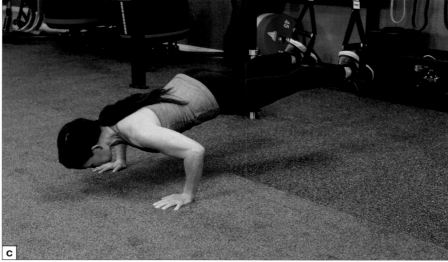

Incline Chest Press With Dumbbells

Benefits

The incline press works the large pectoralis major muscles of the chest as well as the anterior deltoid of the shoulder and the triceps of the upper arm. The angle of the bench combined with the ROM of the dumbbells helps to create more shape for the chest muscles while possibly reducing stress in the glenohumeral joints of the shoulders when compared to an incline barbell chest press where both hands are fixed in place on the bar.

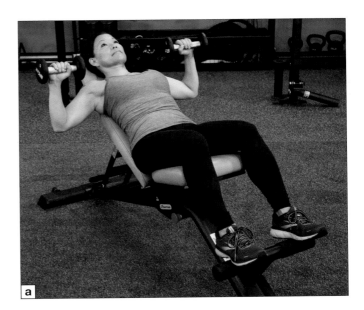

Instructions

1. Use a bench with a low incline (with a higher incline, the chest will be less involved; a lower incline places more of the work in the larger pectoralis major muscles). Hold the dumbbells vertically on your knees, and lift your knees up, one at a time, to help lift the dumbbells to your shoulders. With the dumbbells by your shoulders, your elbows should be pointing away from your body (the right arm in the direction of three o'clock, the left arm in the direction of nine o'clock) but angled down toward the floor.

2. Keep your elbows wide, your wrists in line with your elbows, and feet planted firmly on the floor or footrest (your feet help create stability for the rest of your body; a). Press your hands up, bring them together over the middle of your chest, and pause while squeezing your chest muscles. Slowly lower your arms back to the starting position.

Correct Your Form

When lowering, bring your elbows down only as far as your chest. Taking them too low could create too much strain on the rotator cuff muscles of the shoulder. For safety, avoid going to fatigue. When using heavier weights or working to the point of fatigue, use a spotter.

Barbell Variation

The difference between using a barbell and using dumbbells is that the dumbbells allow a natural, curvilinear motion of the shoulder joints while a barbell keeps the hands locked in place on the bar. Dumbbells allow a greater ROM, while a barbell could allow you to lift more weight.

When using a barbell, place the hands wide so that the wrists are directly in line with the elbows when lifting the bar off the rack. Slowly bring the bar down, but stop before touching the chest (b). Keep your feet pressed into the floor or footrest for optimal stability and control during the lift.

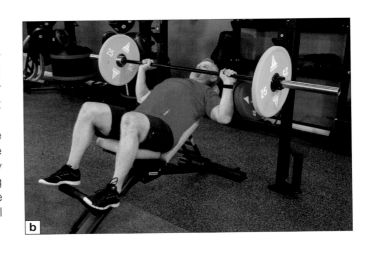

Floor Chest Press With Dumbbells

Benefits

Doing chest presses on the floor might not seem effective, but when using heavier dumbbells, allowing the weights to lower too close to the chest causing the elbows to bend beyond 90 degrees could place unnecessary strain on the rotator cuff muscles as well as the tendons that connect the biceps to the shoulder blades and be a potential mechanism for injury. When you do chest presses on the floor, the elbows can't bend beyond 90 degrees because the floor stops them, which acts as a safety mechanism for the shoulders when a heavier weight is used. Plus, when working out at home, lying on the floor means you do not have to purchase (and store) a bench.

Instructions

1. Lie supine (faceup) with your feet flat on the floor and your knees bent. Hold one dumbbell in each hand with your elbows out to the sides of your body and your wrists directly over your elbows (your elbows should be bent at 90 degrees; *a*).
2. Press the weights up, bringing your hands close together over the center of your chest.
3. Pause and squeeze your chest muscles before lowering the weights back to the starting position.

Correct Your Form

Use a weight that makes the assigned number of reps challenging, but do not go too heavy or work to the point of fatigue unless you have a spotter to help. Keep your feet flat on the floor; pushing them down while doing the lift could help increase overall stability. Exhale as you push the weight up and bring your arms together; inhale as you lower the weights.

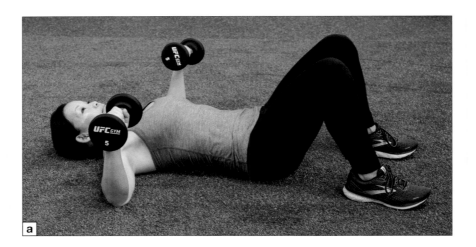

Alternating Arm Variation

If you are exercising at home with only one set of weights, one way to make this exercise more challenging is by moving one arm at a time. Hold both arms straight up in the air, and then slowly lower your right arm while keeping the left arm extended. Return the right arm to the top of the movement, and then slowly lower the left. Keeping one arm straight while lowering the other will increase the time under tension (TUT), which could help recruit more muscle fibers.

Kettlebells Variation

Hold two kettlebells in a racked position (gripping the handles tightly with the bells resting against your forearms) and follow the dumbbell instructions (b). Holding the kettlebells in this position requires a lot of grip and forearm strength. When first performing this movement, use kettlebells that are lighter than the dumbbells you normally use. Improving your grip and forearm strength could help you to more easily and efficiently perform a number of ADLs.

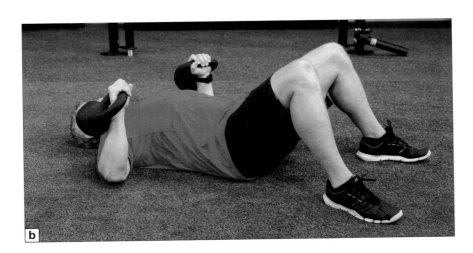

One-Arm Cable Chest Press

Benefits

Pushing from one side of your body can help engage the deep muscles responsible for stabilizing your spine. In addition, chest presses from a standing position allow for a greater ROM from the shoulder than normal chest presses on a hard bench, which can restrict motion of the shoulder blade.

Instructions

1. Set the pulley of a cable machine at approximately chest height. Stand facing away from the anchor point, and grip the handle tightly in your hand so that the cable is directly on top of your forearm. Your elbow should be directly in line with the pulley.
2. Keep your feet shoulder-width apart and your left foot slightly forward (the heel of the left foot should be even with the toes of your right). Keeping your pelvis level, press your feet into the ground to activate the muscles that stabilize your spine.
3. Keeping your spine tall, press your right arm forward. Pause at the end for 2 to 3 seconds before slowly bringing your arm back to the starting position.

Correct Your Form

For optimal ROM from your shoulder, keep your spine long and lift your chest as you press your arm forward. If the cable is moving over your shoulder or arm, make sure your elbow is directly in front of the cable pulley.

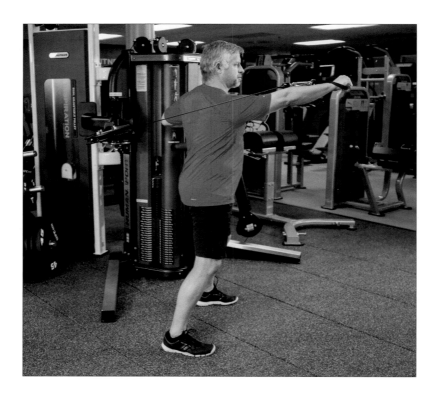

One-Arm Overhead Press
With Dumbbell

Benefits

The one-arm overhead press uses your hip, arm, shoulder, forearm, and grip muscles with one move that is a true test of strength. Unilateral exercises can help develop more strength because they focus all of your energy into the working muscles. In addition, lifting with one arm at a time requires the muscles that stabilize the spine to work harder, which can help develop a stronger core.

Instructions

1. Stand with your feet hip-width apart so that your right foot is slightly in front of your left. Hold a dumbbell with your right hand positioned in front of your right shoulder so that your elbow is bent and your upper arm is next to your rib cage while keeping your left arm by your side (*a*). When starting, your bodyweight should be shifted into the back leg (the left in the instructions).
2. Press your left foot into the ground to shift your weight forward. As your weight moves forward into your right hip, press your right arm straight overhead, keeping the palm of your right hand facing the midline of your body (*b*).
3. Think about pulling your right elbow back down to your rib cage as you lower the weight.

Correct Your Form

Even though this is primarily a shoulder exercise, the feet and hips play an important role in activating the muscles that stabilize your spine. You start the move with your feet by pressing into the ground and complete it once your arm is fully extended; when lowering the weight, pull your elbow back down toward your rib cage. Keep your spine long and tall so that you have an optimal ROM from your shoulder joint. Control the downward motion by pulling the elbow down rather than just letting the weight fall.

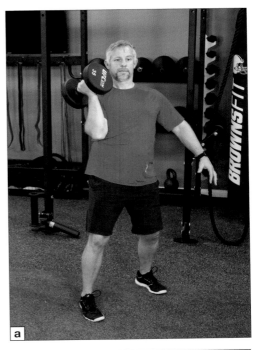

a

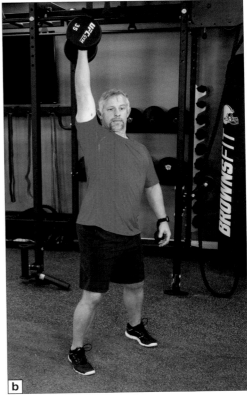

b

Kettlebell Racked Variation

Hold the kettlebell in your right hand so the fingertips of your right hand are by your right collarbone and your right elbow is next to your rib cage with the kettlebell resting on your forearm (c). As you press the kettlebell overhead, allow your arm to rotate so that your palm is facing the middle of your body at the top of the movement.

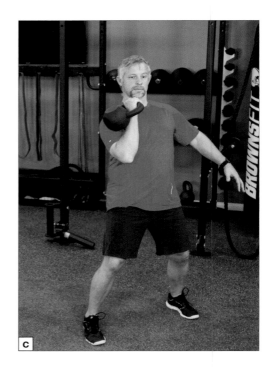

Kettlebell Bottom-Up Variation

Holding the kettlebell in an inverted position requires more grip strength, which helps to engage more shoulder muscles. Hold the kettlebell by the handle so that the bottom is facing the ceiling and repeat the steps from the dumbbell instructions (d). Note that this requires a lot of grip strength. When first performing this exercise, use a lighter weight than normal to help develop your forearm, wrist, and hand muscles.

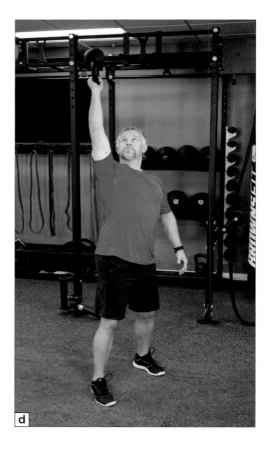

Standing Shoulder Press With Dumbbells

Benefits

The scapula bones that create the foundation for the shoulders are connected to the pelvis via the spine. Many of the muscles that connect the shoulders and pelvis to the spine can be considered part of the musculature of the core. Shoulder presses from a standing position involve the muscles that control motion at the hips, making this a total body exercise. This can help to burn more calories than doing presses from a seated position. Plus, doing presses in a standing position can help you to prepare for movements that require the shoulders and hips to work together, like putting a bag in an overhead bin on an airplane or putting an object on a high shelf.

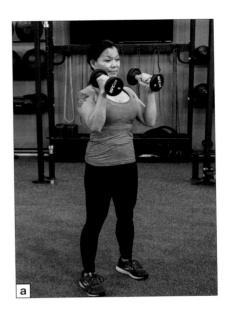

Instructions

1. Stand with your feet hip-width apart. Grip one dumbbell in each hand and hold them in front of each shoulder with your elbows tucked close to your body so that the palms of your hands are facing one another (*a*).
2. Keeping a slight bend in your knees, press both feet into the floor as you press both arms directly overhead, keeping your palms facing the midline of your body.
3. From the top of the movement, slowly return the weight to your shoulders by pulling your arms down from the elbows. This will activate the latissimus dorsi muscles of the upper back, helping to keep the shoulder joints safer.

Correct Your Form

Presses with your shoulders out wide could impinge the biceps tendon. The position described in the instructions is safer for the shoulder joints and may feel awkward at first, but it won't be long before your shoulders are stronger and more stable. When lowering, don't just let the arms fall down; control the motion by pulling your elbows back toward your rib cage.

Kettlebells Racked Variation

Hold the kettlebells in a racked position so that your upper arms are next to the sides of your body, your forearms are in front of your chest, and your palms are facing the midline of your body. The round parts of the kettlebells should be resting on top of your forearms (*b*). Pressing your feet into the ground for stability, press both arms overhead. As your arms move upward, rotate your palms to face each other at the top of the movement. Pull your elbows back down to return the weights to the starting position, palms facing your body.

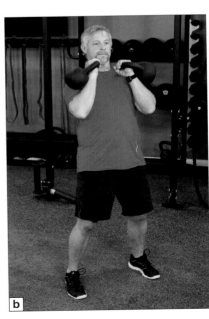

Barbell Variation

Place a barbell on a rack at approximately shoulder height. Place both hands on the bar with a palms-down grip at a little wider than shoulder-width apart. Dip your hips to drop under the bar, and grip it tight as you extend your hips to lift it off the rack. Press both feet into the floor to activate your core stabilizers as you squeeze the bar and press it directly overhead.

Two-Arm Push Press With Kettlebells

Benefits

This may look like a shoulder press, but in reality, it is an explosive lift where the force to move the weight is generated by the legs; the arms and shoulders just guide the movement. In addition to integrating the muscles of the lower and upper body so they can work together more efficiently, this power exercise can help recruit the larger type II muscle fibers responsible for muscle growth, definition, and carbohydrate metabolism.

Instructions

1. Hold one kettlebell in each hand in the racked position so your fingertips are near your collarbone and your elbows are close to your rib cage; squeeze the handles tightly (a).
2. Keeping your feet about shoulder-width apart, quickly drop into a quarter squat before explosively pressing your feet into the floor and snapping your hips forward while pressing both arms straight overhead (b). The hip dip and explosive hip extension of snapping forward should happen in quick succession. As your arms move over your head, rotate your wrists so that you finish the move with your palms facing forward.
3. Control the downward motion of the weights by pulling your elbows down to your rib cage as you lower the kettlebells back to the starting position. Reload in the racked position before the next rep.

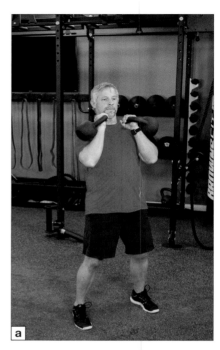

Correct Your Form

Keep your spine straight and feet planted into the floor to create stability and enhance the amount of power your hips can generate; the harder you can press into the floor, the more force you should be able to generate as you push the kettlebells straight overhead. Gripping the handles tightly and pressing your feet into the ground can help recruit the deep core muscles that stabilize the spine.

Dumbbells Variation

Standing with your feet approximately hip-width apart, hold one dumbbell in each hand so that your palms are facing one another with your elbows close to your rib cage. Keeping your spine long, quickly sink into your hips, explosively press your feet into the floor, and snap your hips forward as you extend your arms straight overhead (your arms should rotate slightly toward the front of your body as you extend them overhead). Slowly lower your arms by pulling your elbows down toward your rib cage.

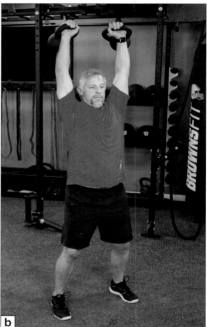

Cable Two-Hand Press (Pallof Press)

Benefits

This exercise is a progression from the front plank, which takes place in a facedown position, to increase the strength and coordination between your hips and shoulders. You will also strengthen the muscles that stabilize your spine; as they become stronger, they can give the appearance of a flatter stomach.

Instructions

1. Set the cable pulley at approximately shoulder height, and stand with the right side of your body closest to the anchor point of the pulley. Hold the handle with the fingers of both hands interlaced.
2. Stand far enough away from the anchor point so that there is tension on the cable. Place your feet shoulder-width apart, and keep your pelvis level, with your knees slightly bent, during the exercise so that you are anchoring yourself by pressing both feet into the ground.
3. Begin with your elbows in by your sides, touching your rib cage. Keeping your spine tall and long, press the handle forward. Pause at the end of the movement for 2 to 3 seconds before slowly pulling your elbows back to your sides.

Correct Your Form

For optimal stability, keep both feet pressed into the ground while squeezing your thighs and glutes. For optimal motion from your shoulders, keep your spine long during the movement.

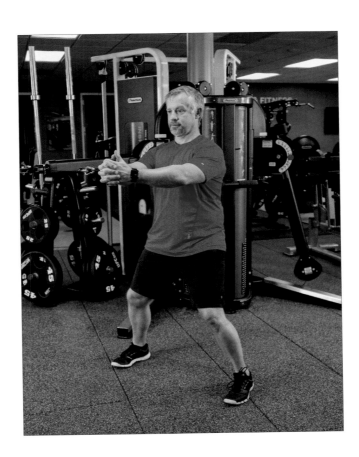

Explosive Push-Up

Benefits

The explosive version of the push-up helps strengthen the deep muscles that stabilize the spine while activating the type II muscle fibers and increasing the rate of force development in the chest, shoulders, and triceps.

Instructions

1. Start in the plank position, legs hip-width apart. Press your hands into the ground a little wider than shoulder-width apart. Press your toes down into the ground while squeezing your glute and thigh muscles (*a*).
2. To explode up, forcefully press your hands into the floor as if you are pushing the floor away from you (*b*).
3. Slowly lower yourself down to the starting position.

Correct Your Form

The focus of this exercise is on exploding up, away from the floor, *not* on doing as many reps as possible. Between explosive reps, focus on maintaining your body position and lowering yourself in a controlled manner by keeping your hands pressed firmly into the floor and contracting your glute muscles. If necessary, modify the exercise by doing the push-up on your knees or by placing one knee on the floor to reduce your bodyweight as you lower yourself back to the starting position.

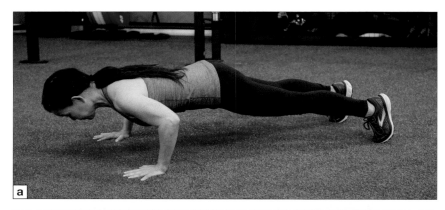

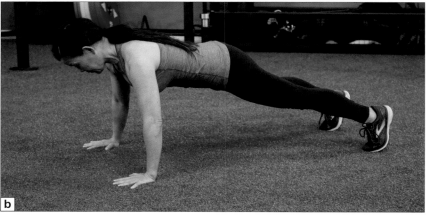

Medicine Ball Chest Press Throw

Benefits

Explosive movements with a medicine ball can help recruit more of the larger type II muscle fibers responsible for generating force, muscle definition, and carbohydrate metabolism. In addition, explosive exercises can recruit more muscle motor units, which helps to develop quicker reflexes.

Instructions

1. You will need a partner, a reinforced wall sturdy enough to sustain the impact of a medicine ball, or an appropriate target like a medicine ball rebounder. A rebounder is like a mini-trampoline designed for medicine ball throws; if using one, stand farther back because the elastic recoil will accelerate the ball back to you rapidly.
2. Hold a medicine ball in front of the center of your chest with both hands.
3. Keep your feet hip-width apart as you quickly dip your hips. Explosively press both feet into the floor while extending your arms straight in front of you to throw the ball.
4. Keep both arms extended with your hands out in front of you to catch the ball, which will be coming back at you quickly.

Correct Your Form

The goal is to enhance the speed of muscle action, which requires using a lighter weight (a heavier medicine ball will result in a slower movement). When starting this exercise, select a weight that is approximately 5 percent of your bodyweight. This is a seemingly simple exercise but requires good technique and form to properly engage your chest and core muscles. Keep your spine long throughout the entire movement.

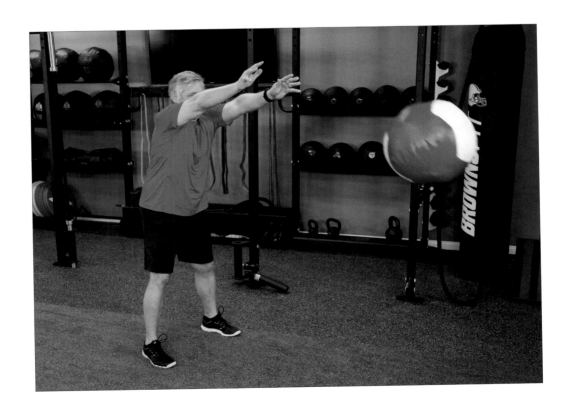

Pulling Movements

Pulling is one of the foundational patterns of human movement and can occur either in front of the body or from an overhead position. Regardless of the direction, the goal is to control the movement as you bring the weight closer to your body. Pulling movements can help improve grip strength while recruiting the biceps muscles of the upper arms.

Chin-Up (Supinated Grip)

Benefits

Using a palms-up (supinated) grip aligns the two bones of your forearm (radius and ulna) next to one another, which can reduce strain on your elbow. With a palms-down grip, the radius crosses over the ulna, which could create strain on the forearm muscles as well as impingement of the rotator cuff muscles (turning your palms down creates internal rotation at the glenohumeral joint). In addition, a palms-up grip recruits the larger biceps muscles of the upper arms.

Instructions

1. Grab a fixed bar tightly with both hands and your feet approximately hip-width apart. If necessary, use a bench or step to reach a high bar.
2. Take the weight off your legs by stepping off the bench or bending the knees so your feet are off the floor.
3. Keeping your elbows facing away from you and your spine long, pull your chest up toward the bar (a). Exhale as you pull yourself up.
4. Pause at the top for a moment before inhaling as you lower back to the starting position.

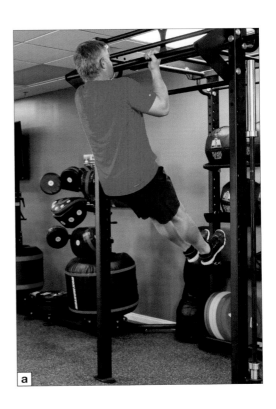

Correct Your Form

Keep your chest lifted so that your spine remains straight and long. Avoid holding your breath; exhaling as you pull your body up can help reduce intra-abdominal pressure. Perform reps to the point of momentary fatigue.

Power Band Variation

If you're not able to pull yourself up, loop a power band (a thick elastic band approximately 2 to 3 feet in diameter) onto the bar and place one knee on the band. Your bodyweight should stretch the band, and its elasticity will help support your weight as you pull yourself up (b). The thicker the band, the more effective it will be at supporting your bodyweight.

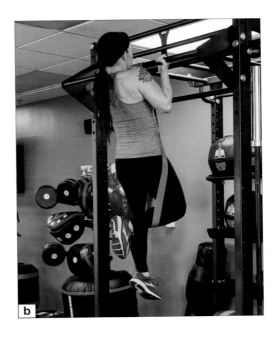

Suspension Trainer Row

Benefits

An important benefit of a suspension trainer is that there are two points of contact: Either your hands are holding the handles with your feet on the floor, or your feet are in the cradles with your hands on the floor. Either way, your core muscles that connect your hips to your pelvis to your spine to your shoulders have to do a lot of work during the exercise to control your body to reduce unwanted movement. Plus, because you can attach it to a door frame, a beam in the garage, or take it outside to a favorite park, a suspension trainer is a great strength training tool for a home workout room.

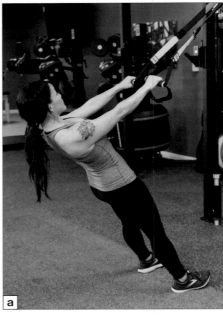

Instructions

1. Stand facing the anchor point of the suspension trainer, holding one handle in each hand, palms facing toward the ground.
2. Keeping your heels on the ground and legs straight, lean back (a). Squeeze your glutes and press your hips forward for optimal body control.
3. As you pull your body toward the handles, rotate your wrists so that you finish with your palms facing each other. This rotation uses the forearm and biceps muscles, helping to improve definition.
4. Keep your body straight as you slowly extend your arms to return to the starting position.

Correct Your Form

The more vertical your body, the lower the resistance; the more horizontal your body, the greater the resistance. If you start to fatigue during the exercise, simply walk your feet back so that you are in a more vertical position. Grip the handles tightly in your hands, and pull your elbows toward your ribs for optimal recruitment of your upper back muscles.

One-Arm Variation

This option can help develop more strength in your upper back and biceps muscles. When using your right arm, stagger your feet so that your right knee is bent with your right foot closer to your body and your left leg extended straight in front of your body. Grip the handle tightly and pull your right elbow toward your rib cage to perform the pulling motion (b). Use your left arm for balance and control by keeping it extended straight out from your left shoulder pointing to the front of your body. Start in a more vertical position for less resistance; as you become stronger, start with your body closer to a horizontal position for more resistance.

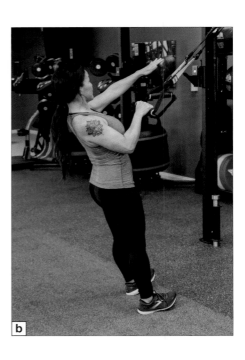

Barbell Bent-Over Row With Supinated Grip

Benefits

The barbell bent-over row engages the large latissimus dorsi muscle, which helps to create the V-shape of the upper body, as well as the posterior deltoids of the shoulders and the biceps of the upper arms. The deep core muscles have to stabilize the spine while your glutes, hamstrings, and quadriceps work to create a stable base, making this an effective exercise for strengthening your core muscles. Using a palms-up grip can reduce strain in the elbows and shoulders while increasing activation of the biceps muscles.

Instructions

1. Grip a barbell with your palms up (supinated) so that your wrists, elbows, and shoulders are in a straight line.
2. Stand with your feet hip-width apart, and hinge forward at the hips to drop your chest toward the floor. Lower yourself until your trunk is at an approximately 45-degree angle. Keep your spine straight and press your feet into the ground for stability. Throughout the exercise, keep your weight back in your glutes and activate the deep muscles that stabilize your spine by pressing your heels into the floor.
3. Pull your elbows back by your rib cage to bring the barbell close to your belly button, pause, and then slowly allow gravity to extend your arms to return to the starting position.

Correct Your Form

To engage the core muscles and increase stability, press your feet into the ground while gripping the bar tightly. Exhale as you pull the bar toward your body, and inhale while you slowly extend the arms. Thinking about pulling from the elbows can help increase the activation of the biceps muscles.

Dumbbells Variation

Hold a dumbbell in each hand so that your palms face the midline of your body, creating a neutral position for the wrist. Follow the barbell instructions for the movement.

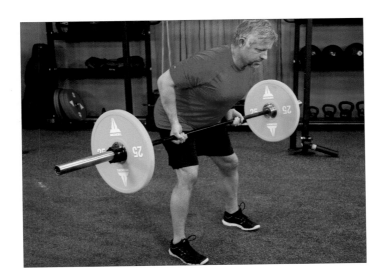

One-Arm Bent-Over Row With Dumbbell

Benefits

Doing a one-arm row in a hinged position without supporting yourself with the other arm can recruit more of the deep muscles that stabilize the spine. This move can help strengthen the core muscles responsible for connecting the hips and upper back.

Instructions

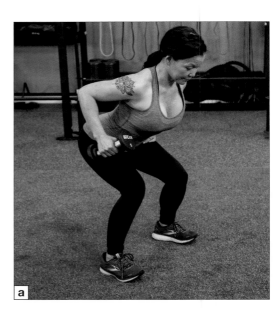

1. Stand with your feet hip- to shoulder-width apart, with the left foot slightly ahead of the right (the toes of your right foot should be in line with the heel of your left). Hold the dumbbell in your right hand next to the side of your body as you start the exercise. Keep your left arm by your side.
2. Keeping your spine long, hinge forward at your hips. Stop where you are leaning far enough forward that your chest is over your knees. Press your feet into the ground to activate your core muscles and increase stability (try not to use your left arm to brace yourself), and grip the handle tightly as you slowly pull the weight toward your rib cage (a). Squeeze the handle with your hand, but think about pulling from your elbow to engage your back muscles.
3. Once the weight has reached your rib cage, with your right elbow pointed behind you, slowly straighten your arm to return to the starting position.

Correct Your Form

Hinging forward without using the nonworking arm (the left arm in the instructions) to stabilize yourself creates an unbalanced load and engages more muscles. Pressing your feet into the ground can help recruit and engage your core muscles.

Kettlebell Variation

Hold a kettlebell by squeezing the handle tightly (a strong grip can help activate the deep muscles responsible for stabilizing the spine), and follow the dumbbell instructions.

Bench Push-Pull Variation

Placing your left hand on a bench and extending your legs behind you while leaning forward can make this a very effective core exercise (b). Push your left hand into the bench while pulling back with the right; this push-pull action can help recruit more core muscles.

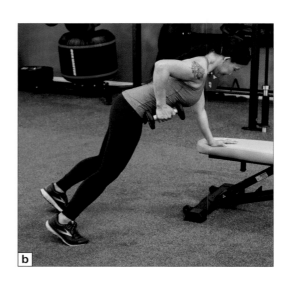

Supine Pullover With Dumbbells

Benefits

Lying on the ground in a supine (faceup) position for the pullover places the spine in a lengthened, neutral position, which allows for a greater ROM from the shoulder joints. If you experience low back pain or the bent-over row causes discomfort in your back, this is an excellent option for strengthening the upper back while keeping it in a safe position.

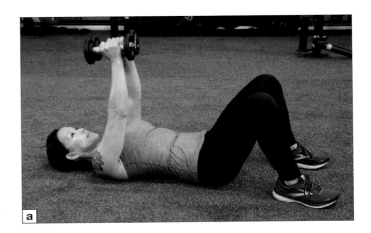

Instructions

1. Lie flat on your back with your feet on the ground and knees bent. Hold both arms straight up in the air with one dumbbell in each hand so that your palms are facing each other (a).
2. Keep your arms straight and inhale as you slowly lower them toward the floor over your head. Allow your arms to go all the way down until the dumbbells touch the floor.
3. Once both arms are fully extended overhead, press your feet into the ground for stability and pull both arms back up to the starting position. Exhale as you contract your back muscles to bring the weights back to the starting position.

Correct Your Form

To reduce strain in your neck, allow your head to rest comfortably on the floor. If a dumbbell in each hand feels too heavy, hold one dumbbell between both hands so that your palms are facing one another.

Kettlebell Variation

Hold a single kettlebell so that the curvature of the bell is in your palms and your thumbs are wrapped around the "horns" of the handle, and follow the dumbbell instructions (b).

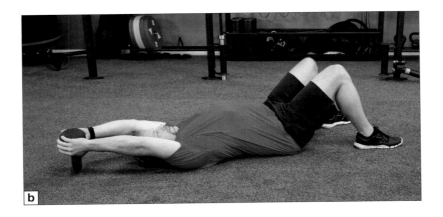

Medicine Ball Slam

Benefits

Slams are an explosive exercise that recruits type II muscle fibers while integrating the muscles of the hips, spine, and shoulders to work in a single action. There are two types of medicine balls: Live balls bounce when thrown against a solid surface, and dead balls hit a surface and do not bounce. A dead ball is recommended for this exercise because live balls bounce back faster, requiring more focus on reacting to the movement of the ball.

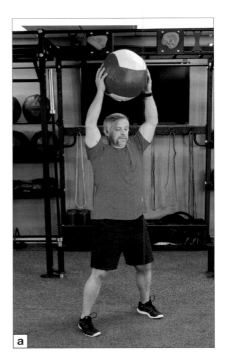

Instructions

1. Stand with your feet hip-width apart and knees slightly bent, and hold the medicine ball between your hands in front of your waist. Quickly raise both arms overhead (a). Then bring the ball down rapidly in front of you with both arms straight, and release it as it passes your waist so that it slams on the floor between your feet.

2. As you slam it down, sink into your hips to generate more force (b). Even if using a dead ball (recommended), you should be slamming it down with enough force that it bounces off the ground, allowing you to catch the ball on its way back up and quickly bring it back to the overhead position. You should feel this exercise in the muscles of your upper back.

Correct Your Form

Keep your arms straight as you lift the ball overhead and slam it down. This will keep all of the work in the back muscles rather than the triceps muscles of your upper arms. Sinking into your hips as you slam the ball allows you to apply more energy to the move.

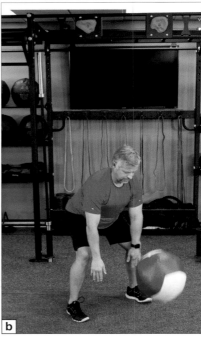

Lunge Variation

If you can't slam a ball, the lateral lunge with overhead lift can provide similar work for the upper back muscles:

1. Start holding a medicine ball over your head with your feet hip-width apart. Lunge to your right with your right foot, keeping your left foot planted into the ground. As your right foot hits the ground, push your right hip back and bring the medicine ball down (under control) toward the ground.

2. Press your right foot into the ground to return to standing as you raise the medicine ball back over your head so that it is directly overhead when you are in a tall, standing position.

3. Alternate side to side, and do the same number of reps on each side.

Rotation

Muscles in the human body are aligned to make the gait cycle of walking or running as efficient as possible. Because the shoulders counterrotate over the trunk when gait occurs, rotational movements are one of the most important patterns to strengthen with exercise. Rotational and multiplanar movements are best performed with bodyweight or light resistance. Heavy resistance should be used with linear movements where the body can generate the greatest amount of force. The movements featured in this section are for heavy resistance or explosive power exercises; for more rotational movements, see the mobility exercises that begin on page 82.

Diagonal High-to-Low Cable Chop

Benefits

When humans walk, the core muscles are lengthened as the shoulders rotate over the hips. This rotational movement with a small squat is effective for strengthening the hip, core, and shoulder muscles all at once. Using a cable machine for this movement maintains a consistent tension on the muscles, helping to develop strength in the legs, hips, core, and shoulders at the same time.

Instructions

1. Set a cable pulley with a handle attachment at slightly above shoulder height. Stand with your feet shoulder-width apart, so that your knees are slightly bent, your left foot is slightly in front of your right (the heel of the left foot should be even with the toes of the right), and your right shoulder is near the handle of the cable pulley.
2. With your left hand, reach across your body and grab the handle of the pulley on the bottom of the two-hand grip; place your right hand on top of it (*a*).
3. Keeping your spine long and pushing your hips back, sink into a quarter squat with most of your weight in the right hip.
4. Press your right foot into the ground as you pull the cable across the front of your body from your right shoulder down toward your left hip. As the handle passes the midline of your body, shift your weight into your left hip and rotate your trunk to your left (*b*).
5. The cable handle should end up by your left hip. As you return it to the starting position in the same diagonal line, allow your right foot to rotate back to point straight ahead, and sink back into both hips in the quarter squat.

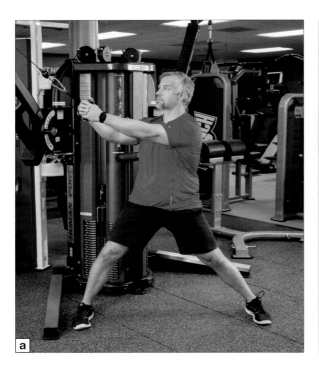

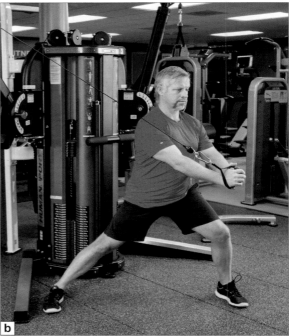

Correct Your Form

When you are starting the exercise, you should lower into a quarter squat with a straight spine. The rotational movement should come from your hips and feet so that the spine can remain long and straight during the exercise.

Medicine Ball Variation

Hold a medicine ball in both hands, and stand with your feet shoulder-width apart so that your left foot is slightly forward. Keep most of your weight in your right leg to start. Bring the ball down in a diagonal direction, from above your right shoulder toward your left hip, while rotating your right foot to point toward your left foot (c). As the ball moves in front of your body, shift your weight from your right leg to your left leg while your right leg rotates.

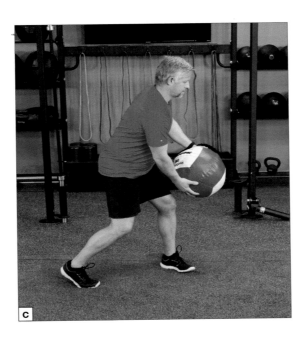

Diagonal Low-to-High Lift With Dumbbell

Benefits

This exercise creates coordinated movement between your hips and shoulders, which is how they are designed to function during the gait cycle. The diagonal movement of the weight demands a majority of the work of the exercise from the oblique muscles (both internal and external), which connect your pelvis to your rib cage in a similar diagonal fashion.

Instructions

1. Stand with your feet shoulder-width apart, your knees slightly bent, and your right foot slightly in front of your left (the heel of the right foot should be even with the toes of the left). Hold a dumbbell between your hands in a vertical position by your left hip.
2. Keeping your spine long and pushing your hips back, sink into a quarter squat with most of your weight in the left hip (*a*).
3. Press your left foot into the ground as you raise the dumbbell across the front of your body toward your right shoulder. As the weight passes the midline of your body, allow your left foot to rotate to the right to point toward the right foot (as if putting out a cigarette someone left on the ground), and shift your weight into your right hip (*b*).
4. The dumbbell should end up over your right shoulder. As you bring it down in the same diagonal line, allow your left foot to rotate back to point straight ahead, and sink back into both hips as the dumbbell returns to your left hip.

Correct Your Form

The rotation comes from your hips and feet, not your spine, which should stay long and straight through the duration of this movement. When rotating the foot as you lift the dumbbell (the left foot in the instructions), think about pressing it into the ground as you shift your weight to the right. When the dumbbell is at the end of the movement over your right shoulder, most of your weight should be on the right leg.

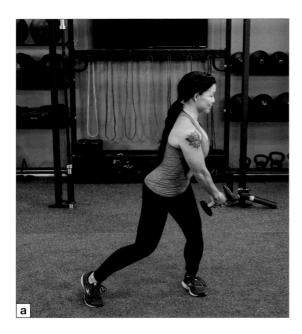
a

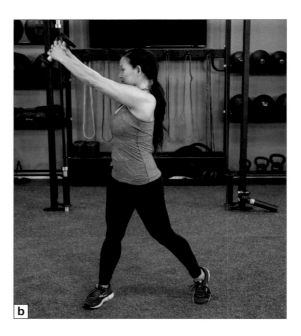
b

Cable Machine Variation

1. Set the pulley at hip height or slightly lower, and stand with your feet shoulder-width apart so that your right shoulder is closest to the anchor point of the pulley. Your left foot should be forward so that the heel of your left foot is even with the toes of your right foot.
2. Reach across your body with your left hand to grip the handle of the pulley on the bottom of the two-hand grip; place your right hand on top.
3. Sink back into your hips to do a partial squat. Push with your right leg as you use both arms to pull the handle across your body, moving diagonally from your right hip to left shoulder while keeping your arms extended straight in front of your body (c). As you bring the cable across your body, rotate your trunk toward the left.
4. Return to the starting position by rotating your body to control the downward motion of the weight.

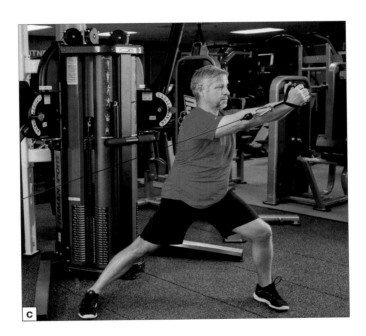

Kettlebell Windmill

Benefits

Your obliques work when you're walking to help control the motion of your thoracic spine over your hips. This move strengthens both the internal and external obliques in addition to the glutes, shoulders, and deep spinal stabilizers to enhance integrated strength between your lower and upper body. Squeezing the handle of the kettlebell as tight as possible helps recruit the muscles that stabilize the shoulder and spine, and also increases grip strength.

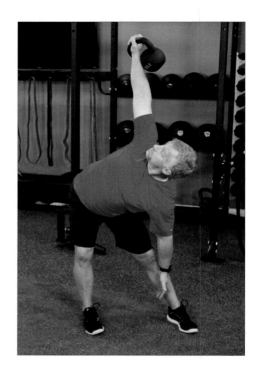

Instructions

1. Stand with your feet wider than hip-width apart so that your left foot is pointing straight ahead (toward twelve o'clock) and the toes of your right foot are even with the heel of the left foot.

2. Hold a kettlebell in your right hand in the racked position: The right wrist should be bent so that the knuckles of your right hand are by your right collarbone and your right elbow is next to your rib cage, with the kettlebell resting on your forearm. Hold your left arm by your side. Press the kettlebell straight overhead, and hold the right arm straight during the movement.

3. Maintaining a long spine, push your weight back into the right hip and turn your head to look up at your right hand while allowing your left arm to drop along the inside of your left (front) leg.

4. Lower yourself as far as you can while keeping a straight spine. To return to standing, press your right leg into the floor and slide your hips forward as you bring your trunk back up straight and tall.

Correct Your Form

It is important to keep your spine straight during the exercise. The movement comes from the hip, *not* the spine. To help maintain a straight spine during the movement, look up at the hand holding the kettlebell during the entire exercise.

Dumbbell Variation

The leverage of the kettlebell helps guide the hip into the correct position. However, if a kettlebell is not available, you can use a dumbbell by squeezing it in one hand to help create stability in the shoulder and spine, then follow the kettlebell instructions.

Suspension Trainer Pull-Push

Benefits

Combining two opposing movement patterns—pushing and pulling—creates rotation through the thoracic spine and hips, which can strengthen hip and core muscles. In addition, the pulling motion with a single arm can improve strength of the upper back muscles that help support good posture.

Instructions

1. Stand with your feet wider than shoulder-width apart facing the anchor point of the suspension trainer while holding one handle in each hand (a). Throughout the movement, lean back to keep tension on the straps while rotating from the hips.
2. Pull your right arm back over your right shoulder while rotating your trunk to your right as you press your left hand across your body (b). You can allow your left foot to rotate toward your right foot as you rotate over your right hip.
3. Pull your left hand back and rotate to your left; at the same time you are moving your left arm, you should lower your right arm to bring it across your body. Rotate your right foot to the left as you extend your left hand back over your left shoulder while reaching your right hand across your body (both arms should be moving at the same time).

Correct Your Form

Keep tension on the straps throughout the entire movement by leaning back; this also helps to activate the posterior muscles, allowing more ROM to come from your shoulders and hips. Let your feet rotate when bringing your arm across your body; they should rotate in the same direction as your hand is moving across your body.

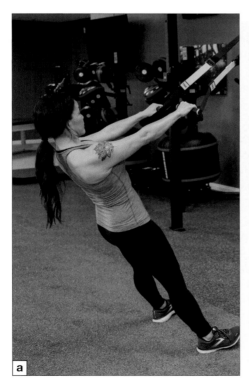
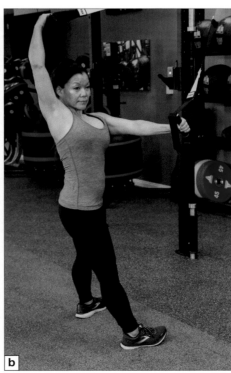

Total Body

While many of the previous exercises may involve more than one muscle at a time, they are based on specific movement patterns. The exercises in this section feature combinations of movements to recruit and strengthen a number of muscles at the same time.

Turkish Get-Up (TGU)—Kettlebell

Benefits

The Turkish get-up (TGU) is a full-body exercise that combines multiple patterns into a single movement sequence. This exercise can help develop total body strength and coordination, and because it uses so many muscles, it is a great calorie burner as well.

Instructions

When learning the TGU, it is essential to first practice the move without any weight to ensure that you develop proper muscle coordination and movement sequencing without the risk of a heavy object crashing down on your skull. Balancing a water bottle on your hand when learning the exercise can help with body awareness and control: You don't want the water bottle to roll out of your hand while you're moving. Practice the half TGU (photos *a* though *c*) first before trying the full movement.

These are the steps for performing a TGU holding a weight (or practice weight) in the right hand:

1. *Pressing the weight into position*: Lie on your right side, and hold the kettlebell with both hands so that your right hand is wrapped around the handle and your left hand is on top. Pull the kettlebell close to your body as you roll onto your back and extend both arms to lift the kettlebell over your chest. Release the left hand and lay it on your left side straight out from the shoulder while you bend your right knee and place your right foot flat on the floor (*a*). Throughout the entire movement, maintain a strong, tight grip on the kettlebell as if you're trying to squeeze water out of a sponge.

2. *Roll to elbow*: With the right arm extended overhead and left arm to the side, lift your right shoulder off the ground as you curl your trunk to end up on your left elbow.

3. *Post to hand*: From your left elbow, press your left hand into the floor as you maintain a straight spine and come up to an almost seated position (*b*).

4. *The bridge*: Press your right foot into the floor as you straighten your left arm and left leg to lift your hips off the floor. Push the hips into full extension while leaning on the left arm (*c*).

5. *The sweep*: As you hold the bridge position with your right foot pressing into the floor, bring your left leg back and place your left knee on the floor. During this phase, your arms should make a straight line from the floor up to the kettlebell to ensure optimal strength and stability of the shoulder girdle. Remove your left hand from the floor as you move into a kneeling position with your left knee and right foot on the ground (*d*).

6. *Kneeling to standing*: Continue to hold your right arm overhead as you press your right foot into the ground and swing your left leg forward to bring both feet next to one another (*e*).

7. *Return to the ground*: Step back with the left leg and slowly lower to a kneeling position. Place your left hand on the floor and move your left leg to the front of your body as you hold the bridge position between your left hand and right foot. Slowly lower your hips to the ground before rolling all the way back to a supine (faceup) lying position.

Correct Your Form

This is not a speed exercise; take your time as you practice the TGU so you can focus on applying strength in each phase. Use your phone or a tablet to record your movement so that you can watch your form and identify areas for improvement.

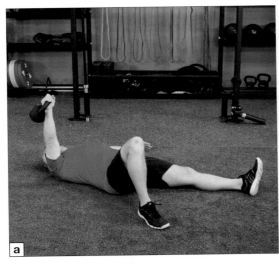

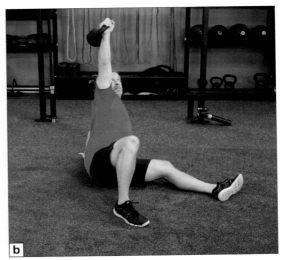

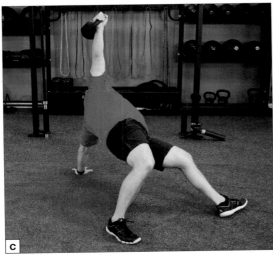

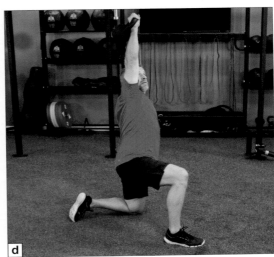

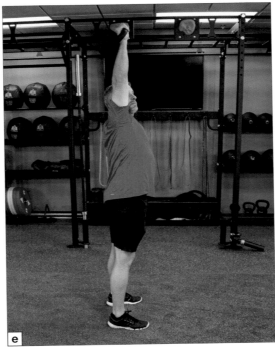

Kettlebell Clean to Press (One-Arm)

Benefits

This is an explosive movement that recruits the larger muscles of the hips and thighs to generate the force to move the kettlebell. Learning how to properly clean a kettlebell so that it rests in the racked position with the arm close to the chest and rib cage can help improve coordination, motor control, and timing. Also, it can be safer to learn how to perform explosive exercises with a kettlebell than with an Olympic-sized barbell.

Instructions

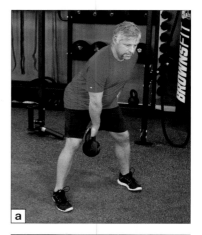

1. Hold the kettlebell in a racked position in your right hand so that your upper arm is next to your rib cage, your forearm is in front of your chest, and your fingers are resting against your collarbone. The round part of the kettlebell should be resting on top of your right forearm. Your left arm should be by your left side; feel free to use it for balance, as necessary.

2. Stand with your feet hip- to shoulder-width apart. Keeping your spine long, push your hips back to start a hip hinge, letting your chest lean forward and quickly letting the kettlebell lower down between your legs. Allow your arm to rotate so that when the kettlebell is at the lowest position, your thumb is closest to you and your pinky is farthest away (a).

3. Once you reach the end of the hip hinge, your arm should be straight, with the kettlebell directly under your center of gravity. Explosively press your feet into the floor while pushing your hips forward. This should cause the kettlebell to travel upward along the front of your body.

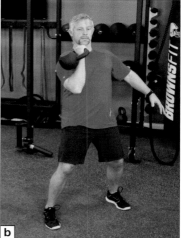

4. Once the kettlebell is at approximately chest height, explosively drop your right elbow and pull it toward your rib cage. As you drop your right upper arm and shoulder underneath the kettlebell (to be able to properly catch it), return to standing in a full, upright position as your palm faces the midline of the body (b).

5. From the racked position, quickly lower the hips and explosively press both feet into the floor to generate the force to extend your arm straight overhead (c). The strength for the move comes from the legs and hips, *not* the shoulder.

6. When your arm is fully extended, lower the kettlebell by pulling your elbow down to return it to the racked position.

Correct Your Form

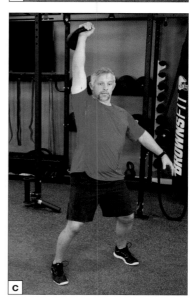

The key to a safe and effective clean is to drop your arm under the kettlebell when it is moving upward rather than trying to flip it over your arm, which is a common and painful mistake. Rotating your wrist so that your thumb is pointed toward you will prepare the arm to quickly drop under the kettlebell to catch it properly. When you snap the hips forward to create the momentum to lift the kettlebell to the racked position, quickly drop your right elbow toward your rib cage as you rotate the palm of your right hand inward toward your chest. This has to happen as one explosive, fluid movement.

Kettlebell Swing Snatch

Benefits

The swing snatch involves the hips and shoulders working together, making this an explosive core training exercise. In addition, it helps develop strength and stability of the shoulder joints.

Instructions

1. Hold the kettlebell in your right hand with your right arm straight so that it is hanging in front of your waist. Your left arm should be hanging by your left side; feel free to use it for a counterbalance, as necessary.

2. Stand with your feet hip- to shoulder-width distance apart. Keeping your spine long, push your hips back to start a hip hinge, letting your chest lean forward and quickly letting the kettlebell lower down between your legs (a).

3. Once you reach the end of the hip hinge, your arm should be straight, with the kettlebell directly under your center of gravity. Explosively press your feet into the floor while pushing your hips forward. This creates the energy for the kettlebell to travel upward out in front of your body.

4. As the kettlebell starts going overhead, punch your right arm in the air while dipping into your hips to "catch" the kettlebell. It should come to a stop directly overhead, with your hips in a quarter squat (b). Stand fully up, keeping your right arm extended overhead.

5. To return to the starting position, first bring the kettlebell down into a racked position, and then drop it back down between your legs to generate the backward momentum to load the next swing.

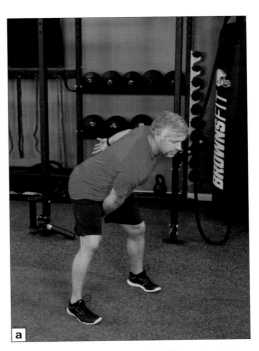

Correct Your Form

Maintain a tight grip throughout the entire movement; the tighter you squeeze the handle of the kettlebell, the more stability you will create for the shoulder joint. Because this exercise requires an extensive amount of strength and stability from the shoulder, it's recommended that you do *not* attempt a swing snatch until you are able to perform 5 or 6 one-arm presses with the kettlebell in a bottom-up (inverted) position. Once you can do this, you will be able to progress to this move and develop a tremendous amount of hip, shoulder, and grip strength.

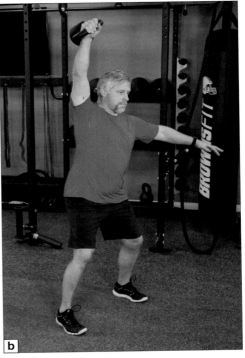

Kettlebell Carries—Three-Way

Benefits

These unilateral movements place weight on one side of the body, which helps to recruit the deep muscles responsible for controlling stability of the spine. Proprioceptive feedback from the weight of the kettlebell places the scapulae in proper position, with an extended spine helping to create integrated strength between the hips, trunk, and shoulders. Both holding a weight overhead and carrying a weight on one side of the body will initiate a reflex, causing the thoracic spine to extend and the scapula to retract and depress. This also creates stability for the shoulder while strengthening deep core muscles.

Overhead

Instructions

1. Grip a kettlebell in your right hand and extend it all the way overhead so that the palm is facing the midline of the body. Squeeze the handle as tight as possible to increase shoulder stability. Retract your right shoulder blade while keeping the arm extended (*a*), and walk forward for approximately 30 feet (10 meters).
2. Switch hands, and return to the starting position with the left arm extended overhead. Next, perform a racked carry.

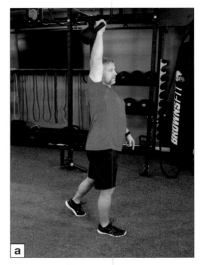

Racked

Instructions

1. Hold a kettlebell in a racked position so that the forearm is close to the body with the elbow near the rib cage and the wrist is flexed to support the weight (*b*). Walk approximately 30 feet (10 meters).
2. Switch hands, and return to the starting position. Next, perform a suitcase carry.

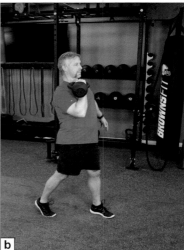

Suitcase

Instructions

1. Grip the weight in the right hand so that the palm is facing the thigh with the thumb pointed forward (*c*). Walk forward for 30 feet (10 meters), switch hands, and return to the starting position.
2. After completing one trip with each hand for each carry, you have completed the entire exercise. Rest before completing more repetitions.

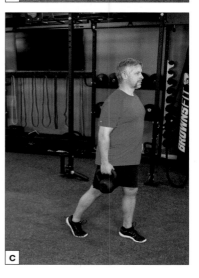

Correct Your Form

This is not a speed drill; the purpose is to develop integrated strength between your shoulders and hips. Take your time while walking, especially when carrying the kettlebell in an overhead position.

Bottom-Up Variation

Holding the kettlebell in an inverted, bottom-up position for the overhead and racked carries requires more grip strength; this helps engage the stabilizer muscles of the shoulder and spine more effectively (*d*).

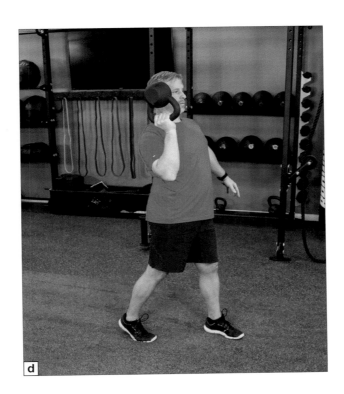

Squat to Overhead Lift
With Dumbbell (Vertical Chops)

Benefits

Fully extending your arms overhead strengthens your abdominal muscles from a lengthened position. This is the most effective method for strengthening the fascia and elastic connective tissues. In addition, because you are doing a squat during the movement, you will be using the thigh muscles and glutes. This strengthens most of the muscles in your lower body while increasing the overall caloric expenditure.

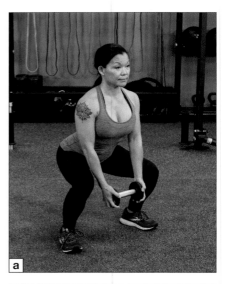

Instructions

1. Stand with your feet shoulder-width apart and your knees slightly bent. Hold a dumbbell between your hands in a horizontal position directly in front of your waist.
2. Keeping your spine long and your arms straight, push your hips back to lower into a squat. The dumbbell should come down between your knees; this should be the lowest part of the squat (a).
3. Return to standing, pressing your feet into the ground and your hips forward as you swing your arms directly overhead, keeping your elbows straight. At the top position, your arms should be directly overhead and you should feel your abdominal muscles lengthened (b).
4. Keeping your arms straight, lower both arms down in front of your body as you sink into a squat (allowing your hips and knees to bend at the same time). The dumbbell should come to a rest between your knees while your arms are still straight and your weight is back in your hips.

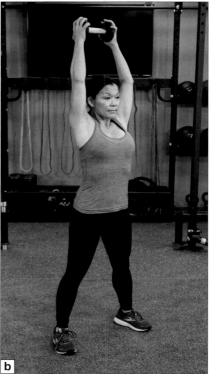

Correct Your Form

The first movement in the squat should be your hips moving backward. It doesn't matter how deep you squat as long as you are moving from the hips first. When standing up from the bottom of the squat, pressing your feet into the ground helps to engage most of the muscles in your legs and hips. Keep your spine long during the movement to ensure that the larger muscles of the hips can do their job.

Resistance Training Programs to Achieve Successful Aging

When considering the amount of exercise that could help you to achieve successful aging, the most important factors are frequency and consistency. In one study conducted among women in their 60s and 70s, researchers compared outcomes of high-intensity resistance training frequency of once, twice, and three times a week. All three groups increased strength over the nine-week study, but the three-sessions-per-week group experienced the greatest increase in functional strength (Farinatti et al. 2013). The 2019 position statement on resistance training for older adults released by the National Strength and Conditioning Association (NSCA) suggests that "a properly designed resistance training program for older adults should include an individualized, periodized approach working toward 2-3 sets of 1-2 multijoint exercises per major muscle group, achieving intensities of 70-85% of 1 repetition maximum (1RM—which corresponds with 12 to 6 reps, respectively), 2-3 times per week, including power exercises performed at higher velocities. Resistance training programs for older adults should follow the principles of individualization, periodization, and progression" (Fragala et al. 2019).

Based on those guidelines, tables 6.1 to 6.9 organize the exercises introduced earlier in this chapter into separate workout programs based on equipment and movement patterns. These workouts are designed to help you to achieve successful aging and, for best results, should be performed consistently for approximately eight weeks at a time. How to organize each of these workouts into a yearly plan consistent with the 2019 NSCA position statement on resistance training for older adults will be discussed at length in chapter 8 (Fragala et al. 2019). The workouts include all movement patterns and alternate in intensity to apply different stimuli to the working muscles. The intensity for each program is written in terms of repetition maximum (RM), which is the maximum number of repetitions required to reach a point of momentary fatigue with a specific weight; *10RM* means that you should use a weight challenging enough to cause momentary fatigue by the 10th rep. If you can do more than 10 reps, add weight. It is more desirable to reach fatigue in fewer reps. If you are exercising at home with only one or two sets of weights, either perform reps until you reach fatigue or perform as many reps as possible in 30 to 45 seconds.

Each workout should include a warm-up using either one of the bodyweight mobility programs from chapter 4 or 10 to 15 minutes of low- to moderate-intensity metabolic conditioning, from 3 to 6/10 rating of perceived exertion (RPE is a subjective scale to determine the intensity of an exercise and will be discussed in chapter 7), to fully prepare the muscles for the work they will perform in the workout. Remember, these programs are intended to help you to achieve successful aging and mitigate the effects of biological aging; therefore, movement-based exercises featuring multiple muscle groups are selected. If there are additional exercises that you like doing for a specific muscle group, like biceps curls or triceps extensions, feel free to add two to four sets at the end of each workout. Keep in mind that these movement-based exercises use a large amount of muscle tissue. When you perform them to the point of fatigue (the inability to do another rep), you will be burning a lot of calories while potentially elevating levels of muscle-building hormones.

Tables 6.1 to 6.5 offer strength workout programs. The warm-up phase of each workout should be about 10 to 15 minutes, the resistance training phase should be between 30 and 45 minutes, and you should allow for a brief cool-down of five minutes or so where you can stretch tight muscles or post the selfie you took while you were working hard. It *is* the 2020s, so it's important to acknowledge that a social media post is part of the modern workout experience.

Table 6.1 Strength Workout Program 1—Barbell and Cable Machine

Exercise	Intensity	Reps	Rest interval	Sets
Barbell deadlift (p. 113)	6-10RM	6-10	30-45 sec	2-4
Incline chest press with barbell (p. 127)	6-10RM	6-10	30-45 sec	2-4
Barbell bent-over row with supinated grip (p. 141)	6-10RM	6-10	30-45 sec	2-4
Standing shoulder press with barbell (p. 133)	6-10RM	6-10	30-45 sec	2-4
Barbell hip thrust (p. 111)	6-10RM	6-10	30-45 sec	2-4
Diagonal high-to-low cable chop (p. 146)	6-10RM	6-10	30-45 sec	2-4
Cable two-hand press (p. 135)	6-10RM	6-10	30-45 sec	2-4

Note: To increase the metabolic overload, the incline chest presses and bent-over rows can be done as supersets, one immediately after the other with no rest; same with the hip thrusts and standing shoulder presses as well as the cable exercises. Supersets help increase metabolic overload and save time.

Table 6.2 Strength Workout Program 2—Dumbbells

Exercise	Intensity	Reps	Rest interval	Sets
Romanian deadlift (RDL) with dumbbells (p. 112)	6-10RM	6-10	30-45 sec	2-4
Rear-foot elevated split squat with dumbbells (p. 120)	6-10RM	6-10	30-45 sec	2-4
Incline chest press with dumbbells (p. 127)	6-10RM	6-10	30-45 sec	2-4
One-arm bent-over row with dumbbell (p. 142)	6-10RM	6-10	30-45 sec	2-4
One-arm overhead press with dumbbell (p. 131)	6-10RM	6-10	30-45 sec	2-4
Squat to overhead lift with dumbbell (p. 158)	6-10RM	6-10	30-45 sec	2-4
Diagonal low-to-high lift with dumbbell (p. 148)	6-10RM	6-10	30-45 sec	2-4

Note: Once you have learned these movements, you can do this workout as a circuit to increase metabolic overload while saving time. Perform one exercise after the other with minimal rest; allow 90 sec to 2 min rest after all exercises.

Table 6.3 Strength Workout Program 3—Kettlebell, Bodyweight, and Suspension Trainer

Exercise	Intensity	Reps	Rest interval	Sets
Kettlebell carries—three-way (p. 156)	Heavy	30 ft (10 m)	45 sec (after all three)	1-3
Kettlebell goblet squat (p. 114)	6-10RM	6-10	45 sec	2-4
Single-leg Romanian deadlift (RDL) with kettlebell (p. 118)	6-10RM	6-10	45 sec	2-4
Chin-up (p. 139) (option—modify by using a power band to help support bodyweight)	Bodyweight	To fatigue	45 sec	2-4
Suspension trainer pull-push (p. 151)	Bodyweight	10-12	45 sec	2-4
Suspension trainer push-up (p. 126)	Bodyweight	To fatigue	45 sec	2-4
Kettlebell windmill (p. 150)	6-10RM	6-10	45 sec	2-4
Turkish get-up (TGU)—kettlebell (p. 152)	4-6RM	4-6	45 sec	2-4

Table 6.4   **Strength Workout Program 4—Dumbbells and Suspension Trainer**

Exercise	Intensity	Reps	Rest interval	Sets
Suspension trainer pull-push (p. 151)	Bodyweight	10-15	30 sec	2-4
Suspension trainer row (p. 140)	Bodyweight	To fatigue	30 sec	2-4
Suspension trainer push-up with hands on the floor and feet in the foot cradles (p. 126)	Bodyweight	To fatigue	30 sec	2-4
Squat to overhead lift with dumbbell (p. 158)	10-15RM	10-15	30 sec	2-4
Supine pullover with dumbbells (p. 143)	10-15RM	10-15	30 sec	2-4
Standing shoulder press with dumbbells (p. 133)	10-15RM	10-15	30 sec	2-4
Reverse lunge with dumbbells (p. 119)	10-15RM	10-15	30 sec	2-4
Diagonal low-to-high lift with dumbbell (p. 148)	10-15RM	10-15	30 sec	2-4

Note: To increase metabolic overload and save time, this workout can be organized into two different circuits. First perform all of the suspension trainer exercises, one after the other with no rest in between; rest no more than 90 sec after completing all exercises, and perform two to four circuits. Then perform all of the dumbbell exercises as a circuit, resting no more than 90 sec after completing all exercises, and perform two to four circuits.

Table 6.5   **Strength Workout Program 5—Barbell, Bodyweight, Dumbbells, Cable Machine, and Kettlebell**

Exercise	Intensity	Reps	Rest interval	Sets
Barbell deadlift (p. 113)	5-8RM	5-8	45 sec	2-4
Chin-up (p. 139)	Bodyweight	To fatigue	45 sec	2-4
Incline chest press with dumbbells (p. 127)	5-8RM	5-8	45 sec	2-4
Barbell hip thrust (p. 111)	5-8RM	5-8	45 sec	2-4
One-arm overhead press with dumbbell (p. 131)	5-8RM	5-8	45 sec	2-4
Cable two-hand press (p. 135)	8-10RM	8-10	45 sec	2-4
Turkish get-up (TGU)—kettlebell (p. 152)	4-6RM	4-6	45 sec	2-4

Note: To increase metabolic overload and save time, this workout can be organized into different circuits. Perform the deadlifts, chin-ups, and incline chest presses as one circuit, each exercise one after the other with no rest in between; rest no more than 90 sec after completing all exercises, and perform two to four circuits. Then perform the hip thrusts and one-arm presses as a superset—one immediately after the other, resting no more than 90 sec after both exercises—and complete two to four supersets. The cable two-hand presses and TGUs can be performed as a superset as well.

Power Workouts

The purpose of the power workouts is to activate the type II muscle fibers by increasing the rate of force development. Power training should use lighter loads to focus on moving at the fastest speed possible. Tables 6.6 to 6.9 offer power workout programs. For each workout, the warm-up phase should be about 10 to 15 minutes, the resistance training phase should be between 30 and 45 minutes, and the cool-down phase should be about five minutes. How to organize the power training workouts into a yearly training plan will be discussed at length in chapter 8.

Table 6.6   **Power Workout Program 1—Bodyweight and Medicine Ball**

Exercise	Intensity	Reps	Rest interval	Sets
Squat jump (p. 116) (option—use a box)	Bodyweight	2-8	45-60 sec	2-5
Medicine ball chest press throw (p. 137)	5% bodyweight	5-10	45-60 sec	2-5
Lunge jump (p. 122)	Bodyweight	2-8	45-60 sec	2-5
Explosive push-up (p. 136)	Bodyweight	3-6	45-60 sec	2-5
Medicine ball slam (p. 144)	5% bodyweight	5-10	45-60 sec	2-5
Lateral bounds (p. 123)	Bodyweight	2-8	45-60 sec	2-5

Table 6.7   **Power Workout Program 2—Bodyweight, Kettlebell, and Cable Machine**

Exercise	Intensity	Reps	Rest interval	Sets
Kettlebell carries—three-way (p. 156)	Heavy	30 ft (10 m)	45-60 sec	2-5
Squat jump box jump variation (p. 116)	Bodyweight	2-8	45-60 sec	2-5
Kettlebell swing (p. 115)	Heavy	12-20	45-60 sec	2-5
Two-arm push press with kettlebells (p. 134)	5-8RM	5-8	45-60 sec	2-5
Lateral bounds (p. 123)	Bodyweight	4-8	45-60 sec	2-5
Kettlebell swing snatch (p. 155)	5-8RM	5-8	45-60 sec	2-5
Cable two-hand press (p. 135)	5-8RM	5-8	45-60 sec	2-5

Table 6.8   **Power Workout Program 3—Bodyweight, Kettlebell, and Medicine Ball**

Exercise	Intensity	Reps	Rest interval	Sets
Explosive push-up (p. 136)	Bodyweight	3-6	45-60 sec	2-5
Medicine ball slam (p. 144)	5% bodyweight	5-8	45-60 sec	2-5
Kettlebell swing (p. 115)	Heavy	12-15	45-60 sec	2-5
Squat jump (p. 116)	Bodyweight	4-6	45-60 sec	2-5
Kettlebell clean to press (p. 154)	5-8RM	5-8	45-60 sec	2-5
Medicine ball chest press throw (p. 137)	5% bodyweight	5-8	45-60 sec	2-5

Table 6.9   **Power Workout Program 4—Bodyweight, Kettlebell, and Medicine Ball**

Exercise	Intensity	Reps	Rest interval	Sets
Turkish get-up (TGU)—kettlebell (p. 152)	4-6RM	4-6	45-60 sec	1-3
Lateral bounds (p. 123)	Bodyweight	5-8	45-60 sec	2-5
Medicine ball chest press throw (p. 137)	5-10% bodyweight	5-8	45-60 sec	2-5
Kettlebell swing (p. 115)	Heavy	12-20	45-60 sec	2-5
Medicine ball slam (p. 144)	5-10% bodyweight	5-8	45-60 sec	2-5
Two-arm push press with kettlebells (p. 134)	4-6RM	4-6	45-60 sec	2-5

7

Metabolic Conditioning and Workouts

Running, cycling, swimming, rowing, dancing, walking, stair climbing, and exercise circuits—all of these are common forms of cardiorespiratory exercise, what is often simply called "cardio" for short. The heart is a muscle that pumps blood around the body; specifically, it moves oxygenated blood from the lungs to the organs and muscles while returning deoxygenated blood back to the lungs. The purpose of cardio exercises is to perform activity that elevates the heart rate in order to help the heart become stronger and more efficient at performing its function. Along with mobility exercises and resistance training, this mode of exercise is a foundational component of a well-rounded fitness program. But is *cardio* the best term to use for this form of exercise? To find out, let's look at what's happening in the body when you work the cardiorespiratory system.

First, *cardio* is a bit of a misnomer; technically speaking, if you are breathing, you are doing cardio. Muscles require oxygen along with the nutrients fat and carbohydrate to help produce the energy that fuels muscle contractions. Oxygen is delivered to muscles via the cardiorespiratory system, which consists of the lungs, which pull oxygen into the body from the air we breathe; the heart, which pumps blood around the body; and the circulatory system of arteries, veins, and capillaries, which transports oxygen-rich blood to working muscles, organs, and other tissues before returning deoxygenated blood to the lungs to be refreshed with brand-new oxygen. Researchers have found that improving the body's ability to deliver oxygen to working muscles is a key component of longevity; individuals who consistently run for exercise could experience an approximately 45 to 70 percent reduced risk of developing heart disease and a 35 to 50 percent lower risk of cancer in addition to a life span an average of two to seven years *longer* in comparison to nonrunners (Nilsson and Tarnopolsky 2019).

While *cardio* refers to any activity that increases the heart rate to pump more blood to the working muscles, it is the body's metabolism that actually takes the oxygen, along with the macronutrients of fat and carbohydrate, to produce the energy that results in muscle contractions. Protein is used to repair damaged tissues and help produce the cells that ultimately create new tissues. Protein can be used as a fuel when carbohydrate is unavailable; however, that occurs only in rare cases during prolonged exercise (see the Dangers of Overtraining sidebar on page 173), so this chapter will focus on how your metabolism converts fats and carbohydrates into the energy to fuel exercise (figure 7.1). Fats and carbohydrates ingested through the diet are processed into free fatty acids (FFAs) and glucose, respectively, which are then used by muscle cells to produce adenosine triphosphate (ATP), the chemical responsible for fueling muscle contractions. Different levels of exercise intensity engage different metabolic pathways: Low-intensity exercise relies on FFAs and oxygen; moderate-intensity exercise metabolizes glycogen into ATP with oxygen; and exercise at higher intensities uses ATP either stored in muscle cells or metabolized from glycogen without the use of oxygen.

Oxygen is essential for metabolizing FFAs into ATP and can be used with glycogen during moderate-intensity physical activity; the more oxygen consumed during (and after) exercise, the more calories expended. The human body uses approximately five calories of energy to consume one liter of oxygen in order to continue making ATP; the more oxygen you consume during physical activity, the more calories you will burn. Type I muscle cells contain mitochondria, the organelles responsible for metabolizing FFAs with oxygen for ATP via a process called lipolysis. This is the aerobic respiration energy pathway, which produces ATP for low-intensity activity and during rest when you are doing a minimal amount of activity like reading this book.

Because FFAs require oxygen for conversion to ATP, the process can take longer; this makes them an inefficient energy source during higher-intensity activities when energy is needed rapidly. When energy is needed rapidly or to generate greater levels of force, type II muscle cells can convert glucose into ATP either with or without oxygen through a process called glycolysis. The intensity of the activity will determine whether oxygen is required (figure 7.2). During moderate-intensity exercise, oxygen will be used to help metabolize glucose into ATP through a process called

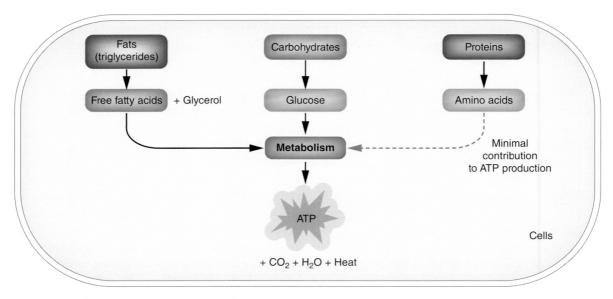

Figure 7.1 Overview of the body's metabolism: how macronutrients contribute to energy production. Energy for muscle contractions comes primarily from fats and carbohydrates; it's only when higher-intensity workouts last longer than 50 to 60 minutes and carbohydrates are not immediately available that protein is used for energy production.

aerobic glycolysis. At higher intensities, when ATP is needed immediately, either glycolysis occurs without oxygen, making it anaerobic, or muscle cells use the limited stores of ATP available to provide the energy for muscular contractions (Kenney, Wilmore, and Costill 2015).

When you exercise, the involved muscles will use one of these metabolic pathways to produce the energy needed for activity, making *metabolic conditioning* a much more appropriate term than *cardio* because it refers to how energy is metabolized whether or not oxygen is required for the process. In general, the purpose of metabolic conditioning is to exercise at an intensity that focuses on using one of the pathways in an effort to make it more efficient at producing ATP.

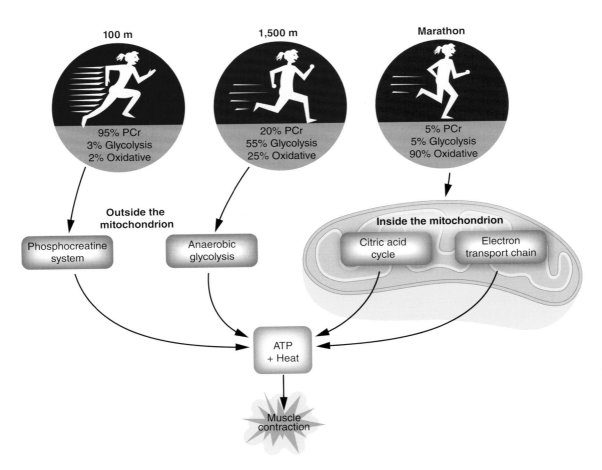

Figure 7.2 How muscles metabolize energy for specific activities. Type II muscle cells have a limited supply of ATP, which can be utilized via the phosphocreatine (PCr) system responsible for supplying an immediate source of energy for a high-intensity activity that lasts for a brief amount of time, like a 100-meter sprint. When exercising at a moderate to high intensity for a period of time of up to four minutes or so, like a 1,500-meter run (it is adaptable based on conditioning), type II muscle cells can produce ATP from glycolysis both with oxygen (aerobically) and without oxygen (anaerobically). One benefit of higher-intensity exercise that relies on glycolysis is an increase in the muscle enzymes that can convert glycogen to ATP, which is important for successful aging. When muscles are working at a lower intensity for a longer time, like when running a marathon, the process of metabolizing ATP from fat molecules and oxygen relies on the citric acid cycle (also known as the Krebs cycle) and electron transport chain to ultimately provide the energy for cellular activity. (Note: The term oxidative system is commonly used to refer to aerobic respiration, the process of metabolizing ATP from fat and oxygen.)

Explosive sports and activities need energy immediately, so metabolic conditioning should focus on anaerobic metabolism, which can provide ATP rapidly since it doesn't require oxygen. The heavy-resistance training and explosive power exercises described in chapter 6 use the immediate energy pathway (the ATP stored in muscle cells that can provide fuel for high-intensity activity lasting 15 seconds or less) as well as both aerobic and anaerobic glycolysis to provide energy. Exercise to the point of fatigue creates metabolic overload, which can promote muscle growth because muscle cells will adapt by storing more glycogen, which also holds on to water, helping to increase the overall volume of muscle cells.

Endurance-based sports and lower-intensity activities like walking will produce ATP via lipolysis and aerobic respiration, which is why low-intensity exercise is often referred to as fat burning. Technically, muscle cells are using more fat during low-intensity exercise, but higher-intensity activities can expend more net energy, making them more efficient for managing a healthy bodyweight. As you will learn, both are important components of an exercise program to achieve successful aging.

Your Metabolism Is Always Working

Almost every large city has a grocery store that is open 24 hours a day. If you need extra eggs, butter, or milk during a middle-of-the-night baking spree because your kid forgot to tell you about volunteering for the bake sale, then you know where to go. Your metabolism is like a 24-hour store; it is always working to burn energy. During periods of higher-intensity activity like exercise or frantically running around your kitchen to make three dozen chocolate chip cookies, your body will burn more calories than when at rest (a calorie is just a measure of energy—the energy required to heat one liter of water by one degree Celsius), but it is always expending energy. How we burn energy or expend calories is technically known as our total daily energy expenditure (TDEE) and can be organized into three distinct categories:

1. The resting metabolic rate (RMR) is approximately 60 to 75 percent of TDEE. The RMR is the amount of energy used to support the functions of the body's organs and physiological systems. The three organs most responsible for burning calories at rest are the liver, brain, and skeletal muscle, which burn 27 percent, 19 percent, and 18 percent of the RMR, respectively. Your brain, the organ responsible for processing information and controlling the body's functions, uses about a fifth of your RMR, which can explain why your ability to think and process information declines when you're hungry.

2. The thermic effect of food (TEF) is the amount of energy your body will use to convert the food you eat into more energy or move it to a location to be stored (as fat) for later use. Eating, digestion, and absorption account for about 10 percent of your TDEE; but no, you can't burn a lot of calories by eating more food. Sorry, it's going to take actual physical activity.

3. The thermic effect of physical activity (TEPA) accounts for the remainder of the energy you expend; it could be anywhere from 15 to 30 percent of your TDEE. Included in this number is the excess postexercise oxygen consumption (EPOC), which is the amount of energy the body burns *after* exercise to return to its normal state.

Unless you are an extreme, die-hard fitness enthusiast, performing random burpees or sprints throughout the day to boost TEPA is simply not practical. Therefore, we have to distinguish between different types of physical activity: the organized, planned activity that is exercise; and the spontaneous, nonexercise activities that occur every time you perform some sort of physical exertion. Yes, exercise is an important form of physical activity that can burn hundreds of calories at a time; however, other forms of physical activity, technically called nonexercise activity thermogenesis (yes, it's time for another acronym: NEAT) are extremely important as well and can play a significant role in helping to maximize the total amount of calories you burn in a single day.

A NEAT Benefit of Being Active Throughout the Day

If managing a healthy bodyweight is your primary reason for exercising, then NEAT is an essential component of that objective. A pound of body fat can provide approximately 3,500 calories worth of energy. Increasing NEAT by 200 calories (about the equivalent of walking two miles) while making healthier nutritional choices to reduce caloric intake by 300 calories (the equivalent of a 12-ounce soda and a small bag of potato chips) equals a net negative of 500 calories a day. If you do that seven days a week, you have reached the amount of calories necessary to eliminate a pound of fat. While a seemingly small step, changing your daily habits by adding more NEAT and reducing overall caloric intake becomes the foundation for long-lasting success in managing your weight. One reason why constant activity is so important is an enzyme called lipoprotein lipase (LPL) that plays a critical role in converting fat into energy. Remaining sedentary for too long at a time could reduce levels of LPL and reduce your efficiency at burning fat, while using NEAT to move consistently throughout the day can help sustain LPL levels, thus helping your body to maintain its ability to efficiently metabolize fat into energy.

Those steps add up; 10,000 steps a day is often promoted as an achievable goal of daily physical activity, but even if you don't make it to that number, adding steps to your day is an important component of NEAT that can burn calories while adding health-promoting activity to your life.

Chapter 9 will discuss specific strategies for adding more NEAT into your schedule.

High-Intensity Interval Training Is Energy Expensive

The classic 1981 movie *Mad Max 2: The Road Warrior* stars Mel Gibson (when he was still accepted as leading-man material; in fact, this was his breakout role) in a postapocalyptic world where a number of armed vigilantes are driving through the remains of society in search of precious gas to fuel their vehicles. In the movie, Max drives a muscle car that requires a large volume of gas; the irony is that Max and the marauders that he battles must use a lot of gas to power their cars as they search for more gas. This is how high-intensity exercise affects your metabolism: When you are exercising at a high intensity, your body is using a lot of ATP to produce the ATP required to fuel the working muscles. Then, after the exercise is done, your muscles continue using ATP to repair damaged tissues and produce more ATP, which is like Max repairing his car when he retreats to the safety of the compound. The good news is that unlike Max, you don't have any Mohawk-wearing marauders trying to attack you while you are performing your HIIT workouts.

Building off of the *Road Warrior* analogy, driving a car (that is, regular driving, *not* postapocalyptic road warrior driving) can provide a relatively accurate description of TEPA; it is well accepted that the stop-and-go traffic of a city can burn a lot more gas than maintaining a steady rate of speed on a highway. However, the constant starting and stopping of city driving can place much more wear and tear on the systems of a car than highway driving.

High-intensity interval training (HIIT) is a form of metabolic conditioning that calls for repeated bouts of short-duration, high-intensity exercise intervals followed by lower-intensity intervals. HIIT is similar to city driving and can be extremely effective for burning calories and improving aerobic capacity, but at the expense of placing high levels of physical stress on the body. On the other hand, steady-state training (SST) focuses on maintaining a consistent, low- to moderate-intensity work rate for an extended period, which is comparable to driving on a highway. SST can be effective for aerobic conditioning and burning calories but can require a lot more time to achieve the desired results than HIIT.

Is one form of exercise better than the other? As with almost all questions about exercise, the answer is "That depends." Similar to driving through a city to get to your destination, HIIT can be time efficient but places a lot of stress on your body. Like taking the highway around the city to get to your destination, SST may take longer to burn the same number of calories but places less stress on the body than HIIT. Both HIIT and SST should be included in exercise programs to achieve successful aging.

HIIT relies on anaerobic metabolism for ATP, which creates lactic acid that can accumulate quickly during high-intensity exercise. The onset of blood lactate accumulation (OBLA), commonly called the lactate threshold and also known as the second ventilatory threshold (VT_2), is a physiological marker that indicates an elevation in blood acidity, which can inhibit ATP production and the ability to maintain high-intensity exercise. When you feel that burning sensation in your muscles, it's an indication of OBLA and a sign that it is time for a lower-intensity active recovery interval. Consistent HIIT can train your muscles to tolerate working at OBLA as well as improve your circulatory system's ability to quickly remove lactate and other metabolic waste. One important adaptation from regular exercise is the expansion of capillaries, the blood vessels where diffusion from the circulatory system to tissues occurs; as muscles increase capillary density, they become more efficient at receiving oxygen and nutrients as well as removing metabolic waste.

Table 7.1 demonstrates that aerobic respiration with FFAs can produce an essentially limitless supply of energy during rest and low-intensity exercise. As exercise intensity increases, the yield of ATP per molecule of substrate decreases, demonstrating that higher-intensity exercise uses more net energy than lower-intensity exercise in the fat-burning zone.

Table 7.1 **Levels of ATP Supplied by the Different Energy Pathways**

Energy pathway	Molecules of ATP produced from molecule of substrate (FFA or glycogen)	Length of time for physical activity	Intensity level
Aerobic respiration (lipolysis)	>100	Limitless	Low
Aerobic glycolysis	36-39	~90 sec-30 min	Low-moderate
Anaerobic glycolysis	2-3	< 90 sec	Moderate-high
Stored ATP (in muscle cells)	1	≤15 sec	Highest

Based on Kenney, Wilmore, and Costill (2020).

How HIIT Became a Popular Exercise Format

On a 1 to 10 scale of the rating of perceived exertion (RPE; where 1 is the intensity of being at rest, like right now while you're reading this, and 10 is the intensity of Mad Max running for his life to escape from the marauders), high intensity can be considered anything over an effort level of 8, while the lower-intensity active recovery intervals would be an effort level of 6 or below. HIIT intervals should be relatively short in length, from 10 to 90 seconds (there is a lot of variability on the exact duration based on existing fitness levels and ultimate fitness goal).

Due to its physically demanding nature and the high levels of exertion, researchers thought for years that HIIT was too demanding for the average individual, and a majority of the research conducted on HIIT was for the purpose of athlete conditioning. Then, in the early 2000s, exercise scientists trying to identify time-efficient exercise solutions for a deconditioned population began studying the benefits of HIIT for nonathletes (Gibala and Shulgan 2017). In an interesting synchronicity, as researchers began validating that HIIT could indeed provide numerous health benefits in addition to the already-known performance outcomes, high-intensity exercise formats like CrossFit and LES MILLS GRIT began to gain in popularity. As a result, HIIT is now a standard mode of exercise in most fitness facilities.

The most limited resource we have is time; there never seems to be enough of it to do the things we want to do, let alone to do the things we *should* do, like consistent exercise. Everyone who exercises shares one common denominator: We all want results from our time spent sweating! An effective exercise program should provide the greatest number of benefits in the shortest amount of time possible. By their very nature, HIIT workouts are designed to push you to your physical limits where you're out of breath and feeling downright uncomfortable. As fitness instructors who teach HIIT workouts often say, "If it doesn't challenge you, it won't change you!" This explains why HIIT workouts have become so popular over the past number of years. Simply put, they work!

The Health Benefits of HIIT

Yes, one purpose of using HIIT for metabolic conditioning is to manage a healthy bodyweight by increasing overall energy expenditure, but there are additional health benefits, not to mention an accumulating body of evidence suggesting that HIIT might be an essential component of achieving successful aging. This means that not every metabolic conditioning workout needs to be a lengthy slog at a moderate pace that is often uncomfortable on joints; instead, you could achieve important health benefits from exercising for less than 10 minutes at a time because when it comes to HIIT, it's the intensity that makes the difference, not the duration (figure 7.3).

HIIT Can Elevate Hormones Responsible for Muscle Growth

Like the resistance training described in chapter 5, HIIT stimulates an increased production of the anabolic hormones testosterone (T), growth hormone (GH), and insulin-like growth factor-1 (IGF-1) responsible for muscle growth and FFA metabolism. Research by Linnam and colleagues (2005) found that "hormonal changes appear to be related to amount of muscle mass activated and to the metabolic response caused by the exercise." Likewise, in their research on sprint interval training, Meckel et al. (2011) found that to stimulate an anabolic response, "input should be sufficient

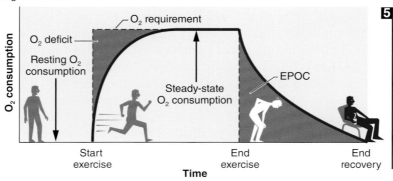

2 Because it takes your body a few minutes to gear up all the systems needed to increase aerobic ATP production, muscles rely on anaerobic ATP production by the phosphocreatine and glycolytic systems, creating an O_2 deficit. This corresponds to the heavy breathing and excess strain you feel right at the beginning of exercise.

3 *Oxygen deficit* refers to how much oxygen would have been used if the aerobic system were able to produce all the ATP from the very second that exercise began.

4 Once your aerobic energy system is up and running, your muscles rely less on the anaerobic systems. You settle in and feel like your body has responded to the exercise intensity.

1 Whenever you begin any physical activity, your muscles have to suddenly increase ATP production from a very low level at rest to a much higher level during exercise.

5 When you stop a bout of exercise, your oxygen consumption (metabolic rate) remains elevated even though you're no longer producing ATP at a high rate. In fact, oxygen consumption can remain above normal resting values for many hours after exercise.

Figure 7.3 An important benefit of HIIT is that your body can continue consuming oxygen and burning calories after the workout as it returns to its normal operating status, known as homeostasis. This is called excess postexercise oxygen consumption (EPOC). Think of EPOC this way: Your car engine doesn't become cold immediately after a long drive; it takes a while to cool down. EPOC means your body continues to burn energy while you're cooling down after the workout.

Reprinted by permission from B. Murray and W.L. Kenney, *Practical Guide to Exercise Physiology,* 2nd ed. (Champaign, IL: Human Kinetics, 2021), 61.

to cause a sizable metabolic effect." Intense exercise *does* indeed produce the results you want from your workout program.

As mentioned in chapter 5, when muscle damage occurs due to exercise, the body will produce higher levels of GH to repair this damaged muscle; like resistance training, HIIT can cause the mechanical overload to stimulate GH production. One benefit of adding lean muscle mass is that one pound (0.5 kg) of muscle can burn about five to seven calories per 24-hour period while at rest; by adding five pounds (2.5 kg) of lean muscle, you could increase your resting metabolism, helping it to burn an additional 25 to 35 calories a day without having to do any additional activity. This may not sound like a lot, but it adds up over the course of a week, and when it comes to managing a healthy bodyweight, every calorie that you can burn counts.

One recently identified hormone, growth differentiation factor 11 (GDF11), may play an important role in how exercise influences the aging process. Scientists have observed that older adults who do not engage in much physical activity have higher levels of myostatin (a protein that inhibits muscle growth), which could explain age-related muscle loss. GDF11 may play a role in reducing myostatin levels, therefore helping to maintain muscle mass during aging. Elliott and colleagues (2017) looked at how HIIT influenced levels of GDF11 and myostatin in individuals in their 60s who were organized into two groups: lifelong exercisers and those with a history of sedentary behavior. Baseline testing for the study determined that the lifelong exercisers had higher levels of GDF11 with less myostatin than the sedentary group, who not surprisingly had higher levels of body fat than the exercise group. The study authors observed that while nine HIIT workouts over the course of the six-week study period reduced myostatin in both groups, it did not significantly change the levels of GDF11 in either group. Noting the effect of lifelong physical activity on

GDF11 levels, the authors wrote, "The correlation between GDF11 and muscle quality is exciting, and may suggest a protective role of GDF11 against aging-associated muscular frailty in humans" (Elliott et al. 2017).

But even if you are a little older and have been sedentary for a period of time, there is some good news, according to a study by Hayes and colleagues (2017): HIIT could help improve the production of free T. The study was based on 22 males, average age 62, with a sedentary lifestyle. The study participants performed a total of nine HIIT workouts on a bicycle ergometer, with each workout consisting of six sprint intervals of 30 seconds each followed by three-minute recovery intervals. Despite having been sedentary for a number of years prior to the study, the participants' total T was increased by an average of 17 percent as a result of the HIIT. The authors observed, "HIIT appears a sufficient stimulus to improve free-T in lifelong sedentary aging men" (Hayes et al. 2017).

Mitochondria Could Be the Key to Successful Aging

In case you don't remember that high school biology class you took years ago, mitochondria are the organelles present in most cells that use oxygen to metabolize FFAs and by-products from anaerobic metabolism, like pyruvate, into ATP. With regular exercise, the mitochondria in muscle cells can become more efficient at metabolizing FFAs as well as recycling the pyruvate and lactate produced from anaerobic glycolysis into ATP (Kenney, Wilmore, and Costill 2015).

Seo and colleagues (2016) observed that mitochondrial dysfunction, a possible outcome of the aging process, could result in a decline of cellular function and the development of aging-related diseases. The authors noted that regular exercise can promote beneficial adaptations to energy metabolism in muscle cells, thereby reducing the effects of aging on muscle tissues. Regarding the role of mitochondria in mitigating the aging process, they stated, "The best target for maintenance and improvement of cellular functions in aging is the mitochondria" (Seo et al. 2016).

Research by Wyckelsma and colleagues (2017) found that over the course of their 12-week study period, HIIT helped improve mitochondrial density in the research subjects who were between 65 and 76 years old. The study authors observed that it is possible to increase mitochondria content of muscle cells even in the later years of life and that HIIT could be "an important and powerful intervention for improving muscle health and function" (Wyckelsma et al. 2017). Increasing the number of mitochondria in your muscle cells could not only help to improve your overall aerobic efficiency but also help improve your cellular function in an effort to minimize the effects of the normal biological aging process.

HIIT Could Help to Reduce the Risk of Developing Chronic Health Conditions

One risk of aging without regular exercise is developing chronic health conditions like heart disease, obesity, and type 2 diabetes; and yes, as with other forms of exercise, the evidence suggests that HIIT could be an important component for greatly reducing this risk. As mentioned previously, when you work at higher intensities, muscles will metabolize carbohydrate, specifically muscle glycogen, to produce ATP; one important benefit of exercise during the aging process is maintaining efficiency of carbohydrate metabolism in the muscle cells. As mentioned, specific enzymes like LPL are used to metabolize FFAs into ATP, and different enzymes are required for type II muscle fibers to convert glycogen to ATP. Research at Ball State University found that adults in their 70s who maintained a high level of fitness throughout their life span had enzyme levels similar to adults many years younger (Gries et al. 2018). This means that performing high-intensity exercise consistently through the aging process could help you to metabolize carbohydrate much more efficiently and reduce your risk of developing type 2 diabetes; because lower-intensity exercise relies on aerobic metabolism, it may not deliver the same benefit.

Hypertension is a common risk factor for developing further cardiovascular disease that could result in an early death. As arterial stiffness increases, it is more challenging for the heart to perform its function of pumping blood around the body. It's widely accepted that low- to moderate-intensity cardiorespiratory exercise can help improve aerobic capacity and reduce risk factors, like hypertension, that could lead to heart disease. It's important to note, however, that evidence is accumulating that HIIT could be an even more effective option than lower-intensity exercise for those at risk of heart disease. In a review of the literature comparing HIIT to continuous moderate-intensity exercise, Ciolac (2012) observed that the former is "superior" to the latter for improving cardiorespiratory fitness and improving numerous health markers that lower risks of developing hypertension and other forms of cardiorespiratory disease.

HIIT has been used successfully to help individuals reduce risk factors for heart disease, and in their review of the research on HIIT, Gibala and Shulgan (2017) found that studies have suggested that patients who have experienced heart attacks or heart surgery could benefit from HIIT as a component of rehabilitation. They also found that other studies showed that shorter, more intense workouts with HIIT could provide more favorable outcomes for heart patients than moderate-intensity, steady-state exercise. In one study, interval workouts were found to put less stress on the heart than steady-state aerobic exercise. In another study that lasted seven years, researchers tracked cardiac rehab patients who participated in both moderate-intensity and HIIT workouts and concluded that the risk of a cardiac event is low for both modes of exercise in a supervised setting. Another study noted, "The results of this randomized controlled study demonstrate that high-intensity aerobic exercise is superior compared to moderate-intensity exercise for increasing cardiorespiratory fitness in stable coronary artery disease patients" (Gibala and Shulgan 2017).

In a meta-analysis that reviewed the benefits of HIIT versus moderate-intensity continuous training (MCT) for individuals dealing with coronary artery disease, the study authors surveyed 12 studies on the topic and concluded that "HIIT is a safe and simple intervention that could potentially be beneficial for patients with coronary artery disease" (Gomes-Neto et al. 2017).

Salom Huffman and colleagues (2017) studied a group of recreationally active women between 40 and 64 to measure the effects of a concurrent exercise program that included resistance training with 40-second sprint intervals at 95 percent of age-predicted maximum heart rate (MHR). The purpose of the 12-week investigation was to determine how sprint interval training would affect the aerobic capacity of the women and whether those who were casual exercise participants could benefit from high-intensity exercise. Researchers observed that in addition to improving overall health, "exercise training programs of high intensity are well tolerated and convey significant aerobic capacity benefits in cohorts composed of older and low fitness individuals" (Salom Huffman et al. 2017).

Many of these benefits are similar to those derived from high-intensity strength and power training, and yes, they are important benefits, but the body cannot function at high intensity all of the time, which is why it is important to perform lower-intensity workouts as well. During lower-intensity exercise, you can help promote recovery from more challenging workouts while burning calories, but without placing as much stress on your body.

Dangers of Overtraining

HIIT, while effective, could have a number of negative consequences that could keep you from getting the results you are working toward. This doesn't mean that you should avoid HIIT; rather, it's a much better idea to limit yourself to three or fewer high-intensity workouts every week because the older we become, the longer it takes to fully recover from a really hard workout. The reality is that our fitness improves *after* the workout, not during it, and if we are constantly hammering as hard as we can with every workout, then we are not allowing our bodies the necessary time to experience optimal recovery.

Higher-intensity exercise *does* expend more net calories per minute; however, exercise at a challenging level of intensity for an extended period could result in the loss of muscle protein when other substrates have been depleted. Muscles have only a limited supply of glycogen; when it is no longer available as an energy source, the hormone cortisol starts a process called gluconeogenesis, in which the liver converts protein into glucose to continue to fuel activity (Haff and Triplett 2016). When protein is used to produce ATP, it is not available for protein resynthesis and tissue repair. If postexercise nutrition does not provide the protein to support optimal muscle recovery, then rather than losing weight from body fat, your body could be catabolizing muscle protein, resulting in weight loss from losing lean muscle, not fat.

Anaerobic exercise increases blood acidity; in extreme cases, acidosis could cause severe damage to muscle tissue, resulting in the breakdown of a muscle protein called myoglobin. If myoglobin accumulates in the bloodstream, it could be an indication of rhabdomyolysis, a condition that can inhibit normal function of the kidneys, potentially leading to hospitalization or possibly death (Kenney, Wilmore, and Costill 2015).

Excessive exposure to high-intensity exercise without sufficient rest periods could lead to overtraining syndrome (OTS). Signs of OTS include reduced immune system function (leading to lingering colds or flu-like symptoms), elevated heart rate, sleeplessness, increased irritability, weight gain (despite exercise), and a significant decrease in physical performance. It can take anywhere from 24 to 96 hours to fully recover from a metabolically demanding high-intensity exercise session. Rest in this case has a broader definition than simply sitting on the couch watching TV. Rest can refer to active rest, which can be almost any form of lower-intensity exercise. If you are sore the day after a hard workout, it may be due to an accumulation of the by-products of anaerobic metabolism, specifically the lactic acid and hydrogen ions related to acidosis. Low- to moderate-intensity exercise the day after a high-intensity workout can be an effective tactic for removing these by-products. For optimal results, make sure that you get a full night's sleep the evening prior to a high-intensity training day and that your next workout is a low- to moderate-intensity session.

If you enjoy high-intensity workouts, continue doing them, but be aware that they do cause significant metabolic damage and that it is essential to allow an appropriate amount of rest and recovery between physically demanding HIIT workouts. Bottom line: Don't stop your high-intensity workouts, but make sure you limit the length of the workouts to 30 minutes or less so that your muscles are metabolizing FFAs and glycogen for fuel, not protein. In addition, it is important to adjust your fitness schedule so that you can fit in active rest days to allow for optimal recovery. These simple steps can help you to safely perform HIIT for successful aging.

Don't Forget Steady-State Training

Yes, HIIT is important, but as with many things in life, while we may enjoy it and it can be good for us, we can't have (or do) it all of the time. If you're not already doing some form of submaximal SST, then you should consider adding it to your current workout program because SST can help muscles become more efficient at aerobic metabolism, specifically lipolysis. There are a number of differences between HIIT and SST; while HIIT does provide important benefits, it is still important to try to do at least one SST workout over the course of a week. Depending on your overall training load and intensity, performing two SST workouts per week consistently could provide additional health benefits.

Your heart is simply a muscle with the function of pumping blood through your entire body; an important outcome of SST is strengthening your heart so that it becomes more efficient at doing its job. Maintaining a steady state in the aerobic zone can help your body become much more efficient at pumping oxygenated blood to your working muscles as well as returning the deoxygenated blood back to the lungs to have the carbon dioxide (CO_2) removed and be reoxygenated (figure 7.4).

SST can help with active recovery from harder, more challenging workouts. Whether lifting weights or pushing out high-intensity conditioning intervals, you can train as hard as you want on one day and then use lower-intensity SST to help with the repair and recovery process on the following day. The lower-intensity aerobic conditioning, around 4 or 5/10, will help remove metabolic by-products while delivering the nutrients that can help repair the muscles used in the previous day's workout. You may be a little sore from that hard workout, but that's when it's important to do some low-intensity SST; once you push through the initial discomfort, you should feel energized and recharged at the end of the workout. You may feel that you're not going to get results from an SST workout because you're not working that hard, but nothing could be further from the truth. And the best thing is that, assuming you do other things for your recovery like proper nutrition, hydration, and rest, you'll have the ability to go back and hit it hard again in your next workout.

When it comes to getting long-term benefits and achieving successful aging, it is definitely better to train smarter than to push yourself to the highest level of intensity with every

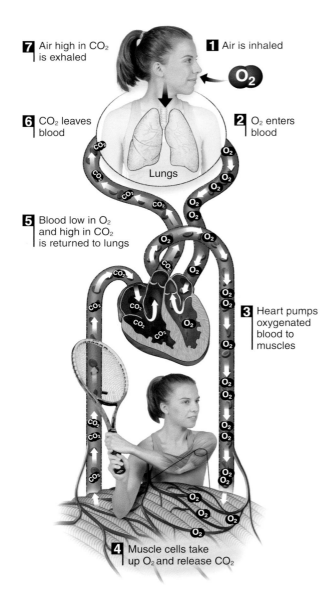

7 Air high in CO_2 is exhaled

1 Air is inhaled

O_2

6 CO_2 leaves blood

Lungs

2 O_2 enters blood

5 Blood low in O_2 and high in CO_2 is returned to lungs

3 Heart pumps oxygenated blood to muscles

4 Muscle cells take up O_2 and release CO_2

Figure 7.4 Lungs pull oxygen in from the air and place it in the blood; the heart pumps the oxygenated blood to your working muscles. Both SST and HIIT can help strengthen the heart so that it becomes more efficient at doing its job.

workout. You can still do your HIIT workouts, but it's a good idea to limit them to at most three times per week and to do them only on those days when you know you will be able to get a full night's sleep, which is a key component of the postexercise recovery and repair process. Properly organizing your long-term fitness program so that you alternate between low-, moderate-, and high-intensity workouts is the real secret to achieving long-term success from exercise. Keep in mind that a long walk or slow-paced bike ride could be an effective SST workout that both burns calories and promotes recovery. Chapters 8 and 9 have tips for how to organize and structure an optimal schedule of workouts for your specific needs.

Measuring the Intensity of Metabolic Conditioning

There is a difference between estimating your heart rate (HR) and identifying where your body is most efficient at using specific nutrients to produce ATP. For years we've been told that finding our target heart rate (THR) as a percentage of an estimated MHR is the best way to determine exercise intensity; however, if you are above 45 and have an extremely high level of fitness, then the HR formulas could provide a rough estimate but lack complete accuracy. It's interesting to note that while the "220 minus age" formula has been used for years to estimate MHR, a review of the research literature could not find any specific source that validates that formula, and many of the existing equations contain margins of error that could be considered "unacceptably large" (Robergs and Landwehr 2002).

Rather than use an arbitrary formula to guess at exercise intensity, consider using the talk test, which can help determine the HR where your body transitions from using FFAs to using glycogen to produce ATP (figure 7.5). The HR where this transition occurs is called the first ventilatory threshold (VT_1); identifying this HR can help you to determine when you are using your aerobic energy pathways (burning FFAs and glycogen with oxygen) and when you are working anaerobically (metabolizing glycogen to ATP without oxygen or using stored ATP).

When you are exercising at an intensity where you can talk comfortably, as when taking a walk or while doing a mobility workout, your muscles are using oxygen to help metabolize FFAs into ATP and you are below VT_1. As exercise intensity increases, energy demands become more immediate, and the working muscles start using glycogen to supply energy. One by-product of carbohydrate metabolism is expiring (breathing out) CO_2, which explains why your breathing becomes quicker as you exercise harder: Your lungs are trying to push CO_2 out faster while simultaneously trying to pull oxygen in. Think of CO_2 as the exhaust product of your muscles using glycogen for ATP—the faster you can push it out, the harder you might be able to work.

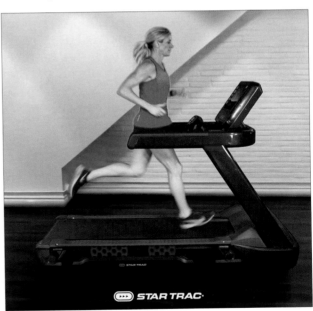

Figure 7.5 The talk test is easy to perform and can help you identify the optimal exercise intensity for your needs.

Once you do the talk test (see the How to Conduct the Talk Test sidebar on page 177 for instructions) and identify your HR at VT_1, you will have the information that you need to design a two-zone metabolic conditioning program in which you can do the hard interval above VT_1 and the active recovery interval below. Developing and implementing a two-zone model for metabolic conditioning can be an effective method of monitoring training intensity while ensuring results. Combining SST workouts that maintain an intensity near VT_1 on some days with interval training where the work intervals are above VT_1 and the recovery intervals are below VT_1 on other days could be an effective way to improve your aerobic capacity without having to exercise to the point of exhaustion.

A second metabolic marker for exercise intensity, as mentioned earlier, is OBLA, where metabolic by-products like hydrogen ions and lactic acid accumulate to increase blood acidity. When you are exercising at an intensity where your muscles are burning and your breathing is so fast that you can only say one word at a time or make grunts, that is an indicator of OBLA—an intensity where you can only sustain activity for a brief period of time before needing a recovery interval to remove metabolic by-products and produce new ATP. Think of OBLA as the redline on your car's tachometer (which measures how fast the engine is revving); yes, when you need to accelerate to merge onto a highway you can push your car to the redline for a brief amount of time, but keeping it there for too long could cause serious engine damage.

Identifying your exercise HR requires using an HR monitor, and while they have become much more accessible over the years (most modern fitness trackers have one integrated into the watch), you do not need one in order to determine exercise intensity. The 1 to 10 scale of RPE can be an effective tool for monitoring how you are exercising based on how you feel (table 7.2). The original Borg scale of perceived exertion used a 6 to 20 scale, which could seem confusing until you realized that adding a 0 after each number produces a scale of 60 to 200, which corresponds with HR—6 (60) is your HR at rest; 20 (200) is your HR at maximal exertion. The Borg scale is used in clinical settings, but for practical application, the 1 to 10 scale of RPE is much more practical. A review of the research literature by Eston (2012) found that when it comes to determining exercise intensity for sports, using a scale of perceived exertion can be a valid method.

Table 7.2 **Rating of Perceived Exertion and Metabolic Markers**

Rating of perceived exertion	Metabolic markers	Energy pathway	Fuel utilized	Length of time at intensity (estimated)*
1 to 4	Below VT_1	Aerobic respiration (lipolysis)	FFAs	Unlimited
5	VT_1 (estimated)	Aerobic glycolysis	Glycogen	3-5 min
6 or 7	Above VT_1	Aerobic glycolysis transitioning to anaerobic glycolysis	Glycogen	45 sec to 3 min
8	OBLA (estimated)	Anaerobic glycolysis	Glycogen	Less than 3 min
9 or 10	Above OBLA	Anaerobic glycolysis transitioning to stored ATP	Stored ATP	Less than 1 min

*The length of time could vary greatly based on existing fitness level; the primary limiting factor is the accumulation of metabolic by-products like hydrogen ions and lactic acid. The more you exercise at higher intensities, the more efficient your muscles will become at removing metabolic by-products and producing new ATP from both aerobic and anaerobic sources.

To optimize aerobic efficiency during exercise, try to work at an intensity where your breathing is quick but under control and you can talk without too much difficulty, which would correspond with a 5/10. A 30-second work interval performed at your hardest level of effort during a HIIT workout would be a 9 or 10/10 on this scale and should be followed by an appropriate recovery interval at 4 or 5/10.

How to Conduct the Talk Test

As the intensity of exercise increases, ventilation (the rate at which we breathe) increases as well. As working muscles transition from lipolysis to glycolysis to produce the ATP to fuel activity, the breathing rate will become quicker to push more CO_2 out of the body and bring more oxygen in, which can limit the ability to talk. Identifying the HR at VT_1 can help you to use a specific metabolic pathway when you exercise; below VT_1 is aerobic respiration and above VT_1 will rely on glycolysis or stored ATP. A talk test is a simple process that requires a piece of exercise equipment like a treadmill, stationary bike, or elliptical runner where you can be consistent with increasing the level of difficulty; a stopwatch; an HR monitor; and a relatively brief phrase, such as the American Pledge of Allegiance or the traditional Happy Birthday song, that you can say out loud.

The steps of the talk test follow; for the most accurate results, it is best to conduct this test with a friend who can help monitor your HR as you progress from one stage to the next.

Step 1: Begin with a three- to five-minute warm-up at an HR of less than 120 bpm or a 2 or 3/10 on the scale of RPE.

Step 2: At the completion of the warm-up, begin the first stage of exercise, which should be 60 to 120 seconds long (it is essential that each stage be the same length of time).

Step 3: During the last 30 seconds of the stage, say the phrase "Happy birthday to you" out loud. Have your friend record your HR.

Step 4: After completing the phrase, increase the level of difficulty. This could mean adding speed or incline on a treadmill or increasing the level of intensity on a stationary bike or elliptical runner; again, to be as accurate as possible, increase the intensity by the same amount each time. For example, if using incline on a treadmill, increase by a 1.0 percent grade for each stage of the test.

Step 5: Begin the next stage; during the last 30 seconds, repeat the same phrase while your friend records your HR. Upon completion of the phrase, increase the level of difficulty and begin the next stage. Repeat this process until speech becomes challenging and you can no longer say the phrase consistently from start to finish without pausing to breathe, whether inhaling or exhaling. This is an indication of VT_1; have your friend record that HR.

You now know your VT_1 HR: If you exercise at a lower intensity, aerobic respiration should provide the majority of the ATP. If you exercise above that HR, your muscles will most likely be producing ATP through glycolysis.

Adapted from Bryant, Merrill, and Green (2014).

Warming Up

Returning to the car analogy, when you hop in your car on a cold day, do you just turn the key and drive off, or do you sit and let the engine run for a few minutes? Letting the engine run before driving off on a cold morning can help ensure that the many parts of the motor are properly lubricated and ready to go before the engine is required to generate the forces to move the vehicle. A warm-up does the same thing for your body: It allows muscles to properly prepare for the physically demanding exercise that you will do during your workout.

Warming up with low-intensity exercise can help increase circulation to deliver oxygen and fuel to working muscles. It can take from 8 to 15 minutes to elevate circulation and improve oxygen flow; be ready to invest that time to adequately prepare your body. An important benefit of the warm-up is elevating the hormones cortisol and epinephrine along with the neurotransmitter norepinephrine (commonly called adrenaline and noradrenaline, respectively, because they are produced in the adrenal glands), which are used to help produce energy by mobilizing FFAs to be delivered to muscle cells, where they are metabolized into ATP. An effective warm-up can help to increase tissue temperature so that your muscles and connective tissue have more elasticity, allowing for easier, unrestricted motion of the joints used in exercise. A good, complete warm-up should make you a little sweaty, indicating that your tissue is ready to work.

When starting a metabolic conditioning workout on a piece of equipment like a stationary bicycle or treadmill, you will want to spend the first three to five minutes moving at a slow, steady pace of about 3 or 4/10 RPE. After about five minutes, as you feel your body temperature start to increase and your breathing become a little faster, increase the pace of your movement to about 5 or 6/10 RPE and stay there for another three to five minutes or until your breathing is quick and you're starting to sweat. Once you are sweating and breathing at a rate that makes talking a challenge, you are fully warmed up and ready for a high-intensity workout.

Another example of an effective warm-up is using one of the mobility workouts described in chapter 4; two to three sets of each exercise should take about 10 minutes and have you breathing at a faster rate, meaning that you are ready for a challenging workout. No matter which method you choose—using equipment or bodyweight exercises—a good warm-up should make you sweaty and have you breathing faster in 10 to 15 minutes.

Getting HIIT Done: Making the Transition From SST to Interval Training

One risk of an extended SST workout is repetitive stress or overuse injuries; one strategy for making the transition from SST to interval training is to switch the type of exercise equipment you use during a workout so that you do not overuse any muscles. When working with clients in a health club, one of my favorite recommendations is to have them change machines every 10 to 12 minutes, which, besides using different muscles, can break up the monotony of SST. Alternating between pieces like the treadmill, stair stepper, rowing machine (figure 7.6), stationary bike (figure 7.7), and elliptical trainer can help the workout time fly by without too much stress on any one joint or muscle group. The goal is to try to maintain the same level of intensity, 5 or 6/10, on each piece of equipment and to try to accumulate a total of 30 to 60 minutes for the entire workout.

Okay, admittedly televisions on exercise equipment seem like an oxymoron, but having a distraction can be helpful. Rather than going to your gym, hopping on a piece of equipment, and mindlessly watching your favorite show, use whatever you're watching to structure your interval training. You want to watch the show, *not* the commercials; during the show, exercise at a level of intensity where you can breathe comfortably, approximately 4 or 5/10, and when commercials come on, exercise as

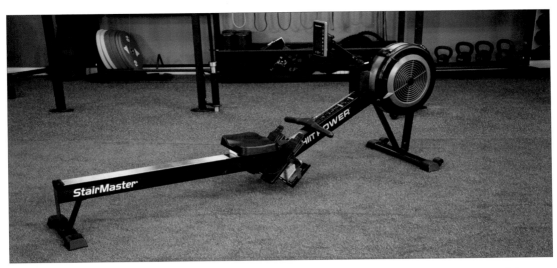

Figure 7.6 Because it uses both upper and lower body muscles, a rowing ergometer is one of the best pieces of equipment for metabolic conditioning.

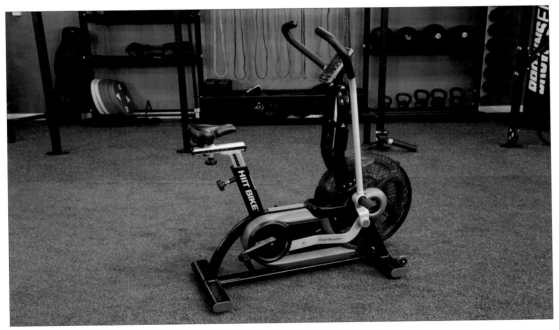

Figure 7.7 Bicycle ergometers that involve both the lower and upper body with the moving arm action are perfect for quick, challenging metabolic conditioning workouts.

hard as you can until you're out of breath, approximately 7 to 9/10. This allows you to enjoy your favorite show and skip the commercials. A normal commercial break is approximately two minutes long, and if show segments are about 6 to 10 minutes in length, this provides a great work-to-rest ratio for interval training: Get out of breath during the commercials, and drop down to an intensity where breathing is comfortable during the show so you can enjoy it.

Rather than jumping right into a high-volume, high-intensity HIIT protocol, it is a good idea to start with a low volume of high-intensity exercise. Research by Dalleck and colleagues (2019) found that a low-volume HIIT protocol, reduced-exertion high-intensity training (REHIT), which features fewer and shorter bouts of supramaximal intensity, could provide more benefits when compared to MCT. The REHIT protocol uses a two-minute warm-up, a 20-second sprint, a three-minute recovery, and a second 20-second sprint followed by a three-minute cool-down for a total exercise session lasting less than nine minutes (eight minutes 40 seconds, to be exact). Over the course of the eight-week study, the REHIT group experienced more health benefits than the MCT group, which performed workouts lasting 30 minutes long (Dalleck et al. 2019). Replicating the workouts from this study would be a great way to start achieving the benefits of HIIT.

Eventually it will be necessary to apply a standard HIIT format like the Tabata protocol. Age should not be a factor that limits your ability to experience the benefits of high-intensity exercise; if you have the ability and the willingness, you can definitely do it. Yes, when done properly, short HIIT workouts can be extremely uncomfortable, but the good news is that shorter bursts of intense exercise could reduce the risk of developing overuse or repetitive stress injuries that could occur from excessive amounts of SST.

The Tabata protocol, named after the Japanese researcher who created it, is a popular model of HIIT that calls for 20 seconds of exercise at the highest intensity possible followed by 10 seconds of recovery, repeated eight times in a row for a total of four minutes. That might not seem like a lot, but when you perform each 20-second bout at your highest effort, four minutes is all you need for a great workout! Note that Dr. Tabata's research subjects were members of the Japanese national speed skating team and were able to exercise at an intensity of 170 percent of their maximum aerobic capacity (Tabata et al. 1996). However, when starting to do HIIT workouts, you do not need to complete the entire four-minute protocol. Instead, my recommendation is to start with a small amount of high-intensity exercise so that you can learn how to tolerate the discomfort before performing longer periods of high-intensity work; remember, when it comes to getting benefits, the intensity is more important than the duration. Table 7.3 provides an example of how to progress to the full Tabata protocol. It recommends taking the established Tabata protocol and breaking it into shorter periods of time so that you get used to working at a high intensity before progressing to the entire four-minute duration. Start with one-minute segments of two cycles of 20- and 10-second intervals, followed by lower-intensity active recovery, and build up to completing the four-minute protocol.

There are a variety of models for applying HIIT other than the popular Tabata protocol. Rather than trying to make one up on your own, consider applying one of the following models. Even if you do not have access to expensive cardiorespiratory equipment often found in a fitness facility, there is evidence that HIIT performed with bodyweight exercises can provide similar outcomes (Schaun et al. 2018). Regardless of the mode of exercise you choose, the goal of each high-intensity work interval is to reach a 9 or 10/10 on the scale of RPE, allowing yourself to recover as best as possible during the prescribed length of time. Remember, when it comes to HIIT, intensity is more important than duration, with the goal being to exercise at the highest intensity possible during each work interval.

Table 7.3   **A Progression to the 4-Minute Tabata Protocol for HIIT**

Weeks	Interval times	Intensity
1-2	Warm-up: 3-4 min	Low-moderate
	20 sec/10 sec × 2 for 1 min	Highest/low
	Cool-down: 2-3 min	Low-moderate
3-4	Warm-up: 3-4 min	Low-moderate
	20 sec/10 sec × 2 for 1 min	Highest/low
	1 min of steady state	Low-moderate
	20 sec/10 sec × 2 for 1 min	Highest/low
	Cool-down: 2-3 min	Low-moderate
5-6	Warm-up: 3-4 min	Low-moderate
	20 sec/10 sec × 2 for 1 min	Highest/low
	1 min of steady state	Low-moderate
	20 sec/10 sec × 2 for 1 min	Highest/low
	1 min of steady state	Low-moderate
	20 sec/10 sec × 2 for 1 min	Highest/low
	Cool-down: 2-3 min	Low-moderate
7-8	Warm-up: 3-4 min	Low-moderate
	20 sec/10 sec × 2 for 1 min	Highest/low
	20 sec/10 sec × 2 for 1 min	Highest/low
	1 min of steady state	Low-moderate
	20 sec/10 sec × 2 for 1 min	Highest/low
	Cool-down: 2-3 min	Low-moderate
9	Warm-up: 3-4 min	Low-moderate
	Apply the standard Tabata protocol of 20 sec of high-intensity exercise followed by 10 sec of active recovery, repeated for 8 cycles (4 min total).	Highest possible during 20 sec work intervals
	Cool-down: 2-3 min	Low-moderate

Table 7.4 provides example formats of HIIT workouts that can be done on most pieces of equipment you can find in a fitness facility. My recommendation would be to use stationary bikes or rowing machines because they are easiest to adjust in terms of intensity and speed; treadmills, stair steppers, and elliptical runners do not allow for easy changes of velocity while working out. For each protocol, do approximately four to six minutes of a warm-up, exercise at a gradually increasing pace until you are sweating and breathing more quickly than normal, and then start the protocol.

When it comes to metabolic conditioning to achieve successful aging, you can alter the types of exercise you do, slow down the pace, or change the length of the workouts. The one rule is to never stop.

Table 7.4 **Sample HIIT Workout Formats**

Protocol	Directions
30:30	30 sec of high-intensity exercise at a 9 or 10/10 on the scale of RPE, followed by 30 sec of lower-intensity exercise at a 4 to 6/10
	After a warm-up, start with five min, and gradually progress to 10 minutes.
30:20:10 (based on research known as the Copenhagen protocol)	30 sec of low intensity 4 or 5/10, followed immediately by 20 sec of moderate intensity 5 to 7/10, then transition right away to 10 sec of highest intensity 9 or 10/10
	As soon as you finish the highest intensity, return back to the 30 sec low-intensity interval; repeat for five min at a time.
	Start with one five-min block; to progress to a second and ultimately a third block of activity, allow for two to four min of active rest, fully recovering your breathing rate between the five-min segments.
Ladders: 20:40/30:30/40:20 40:20/30:30/20:40	In a ladder, a one-min interval is broken up into two segments: one high intensity and one low intensity. For example, 20 sec of high intensity followed by 40 sec of low intensity; 30 sec of high intensity followed by 30 sec of recovery; and finally, 40 sec of high intensity followed by 20 sec of active recovery. After climbing the ladder, reverse the order of the intervals to finish the set: 40:20, 30:30, and finally 20:40 (high intensity:low intensity).

Based on Gunnarson and Bangsbo (2012).

Metabolic Conditioning Workouts to Achieve Successful Aging

Table 7.5 lists examples of HIIT workouts that can be done on most equipment in a fitness facility. Stationary bikes with the moving arms, often called HIIT bikes, and rowing machines are highly recommended and preferred because they are ergometers. This means that the faster you move, the greater the resistance, making it easier to change speeds for interval training. Ergometers measure the amount of work performed either in the number of calories expended during an interval or via the wattage produced while exercising. In both cases, these numbers can be used to track progress and provide motivation; for example, measuring the number of calories burned or the amount of wattage produced during a time interval and trying to meet or beat it in following intervals. The first time on an ergometer you may only produce 50 watts during a 20-second interval; as your fitness improves, you will be able to achieve a higher wattage in the same amount of time. In addition, because both upper and lower body muscles are working, you'll burn more calories. Self-powered treadmills, where the running pace of the user determines the speed of the treadmill belt, are another option, especially for the longer intervals. Additional equipment options include jump ropes and heavy ropes, especially for the shorter interval periods. Finally, bodyweight exercises, like the ones in table 7.5, are always an option for HIIT when other equipment is not available. Powered treadmills, stair steppers, and elliptical runners are not recommended because they do not allow for easy transitions between speeds. For each protocol, do approximately four to six minutes of a warm-up—exercise at a gradually increasing pace until you are sweating and breathing more quickly than normal—and then start the protocol. Other options include performing the protocol at the end of a strength workout or after a lower-intensity fitness class. Keep in mind that your focus should be on intensity, not duration—the research consistently shows that only brief workouts are necessary for great results.

Table 7.5 **HIIT Workout Protocol Options**

Protocol	Equipment	Bodyweight exercises
Tabata 20 sec of work (9 or 10/10) followed by 10 sec of recovery (4 or 5/10) for 8 cycles in 4 min	• HIIT bike • Rowing machine • Heavy rope • Jump rope	Circuit of • Jumping jacks • Push-ups • Squat jumps • Ice skaters
Modified Tabata 4 cycles (2 min) of a Tabata interval, then 1 min of steady state, then final 4 cycles	• HIIT bike • Rowing machine	Circuit of • Jumping jacks • Walking or running in place • Fast squats • Ice skaters
30:30 1 min intervals where the first 30 sec is high intensity (9 or 10/10 RPE) and the second 30 sec is low intensity (4 or 5/10 RPE) Repeat for a total of 5-10 min.	• HIIT bike • Rowing machine • Self-powered treadmill • Heavy rope and jump rope (alternate between 30 sec of heavy rope for upper body and 30 sec of jump rope for lower body)	Alternate • Squat jumps and high planks (30 sec each) • Ice skaters and jogging in place • Explosive push-ups and reverse lunges • Jumping jacks and bodyweight squats
30:20:10 A series of 1 min intervals that are structured as: • 30 sec easy (4 or 5/10) • 20 sec hard (6 or 7/10) • 10 sec really hard (9 or 10/10) This is a continuous cycle of exercise repeated for 5 min, which is one set. After completing one 5 min set, rest for 2-3 min. Then perform another set.	• HIIT bike • Rowing machine • Self-powered treadmill	Circuit of • Squats - slow:squats - fast:squat jumps • Plank:push-ups - slow:push-ups - fast • Lateral lunges - slow:lateral lunges - fast:explosive ice skaters
Ladder A series of 1 min intervals that alternate between a period of high intensity and low intensity within each minute. • 20:40 = 20 sec of high intensity, 40 sec of low intensity • 20:40/30:30/40:20 = climbing up the ladder (the high-intensity intervals are getting longer) • 40:20/30:30/20:40 = climbing down the ladder (the high-intensity intervals are getting shorter) Climbing up and down the ladder results in 6 min of exercise that will leave you sweaty.	• HIIT bike • Rowing machine • Self-powered treadmill • Heavy rope • Jump rope	Complete one exercise moving as fast as possible during the 1 min work interval, then rest during the remainder of the minute. • Squats • Jumping jacks • Push-ups

Steady-state options for metabolic conditioning workouts include holding the same pace or work rate for an extended period of time in an effort to engage the aerobic energy pathways. Running outdoors or on a treadmill, using an elliptical runner or stationary bike, or going for a vigorous hike are all examples of workouts that engage the aerobic energy pathways.

As with resistance training, the important thing for metabolic conditioning workouts is to change the intensity and duration on a consistent basis. When following a three-day rotation, which alternates between strength or power training on the first day, bodyweight exercises on the second day, and metabolic conditioning on the third day (explained in detail in chapter 8), then in one three-day rotation you would do a HIIT workout at the highest intensity possible and on the next three-day rotation you would do a lower-intensity metabolic conditioning workout. Yes, metabolic conditioning can help burn calories, but the real purpose is to improve the efficiency with which your body's metabolism converts the food you eat into the energy that makes you move, making it important to alternate the energy pathways used when you exercise.

PART III

Plan for Longevity

8

Design Your Workout Plan

Heraclitus, a philosopher in ancient Greece, once remarked that change is the only constant in life. Some people enjoy a variety of different experiences in life, whereas others prefer consistency and want to avoid change at all costs. Change disrupts the normal flow of life, which can be unsettling but also provide much-needed growth. When change does occur, it causes us to evaluate what we're doing and consider if we are truly on the right course for where we want to ultimately end up. Change is an important variable when it comes to exercise because too much or too little could keep you from getting the results you want.

What *Caddyshack* Can Teach Us About Exercise

If you grew up or came of age during the 1980s, you are no doubt familiar with a number of movies that may have lacked artistic appeal but made up for it with humor and memorable lines worth repeating. *Caddyshack* is one of those movies, and if you're like a lot of us from that era, you will probably watch a few minutes of it once in a while when you're flipping channels in search of some mindless entertainment. Full of comedy stars like Chevy Chase, Bill Murray, and the late Rodney Dangerfield, the movie boasts many classic lines that have become common sayings. As entertaining as *Caddyshack* may be, the fact is that as you learn the lines, the movie will still provide chuckles but is not nearly as entertaining because you know exactly what is going to happen and when. This provides a good analogy for how the human body adapts to exercise; the more often you perform a particular exercise routine at the same intensity or for the same duration, the more your body will become familiar with the physiological stimulus. It could stop experiencing changes, what you might call a plateau but technically referred to as accommodation.

Change can be a double-edged sword when it comes to exercise: If you don't change your workouts, then they could stop having the desired effect; but if you change exercises too frequently, then your muscles won't receive the stimulus required to make adaptations. After a certain period, the body adapts to the physical demands of the workout and stops making changes. Doing the same thing repeatedly with the expectation of different results is one definition of insanity; the longer you perform the same program, the greater the risk you take of hitting a plateau. This is an important sign that it's time to change what you are doing and challenge your body with a different exercise program.

On the other hand, changing workouts too often or doing different types of exercise with every workout in search of elusive results—what might be referred to as program hopping—is unfortunately a common mistake. Over my (many) years of working in health clubs, I have often seen club members switch from trends like high-intensity workouts to kickboxing to indoor cycling to yoga to Pilates to Zumba to CrossFit and back to indoor cycling. And that doesn't even take into account all of the late-night TV fitness product purchases they probably have lying around in the garage or the back of a closet.

Program hoppers face a different challenge from those who have been doing the same *Caddyshack* workouts since that movie was first released in the theaters. Program hoppers become easily distracted and are always looking for the newest, latest, greatest fad that promises quick results. If this is you, here's an important secret about exercise: it doesn't matter what type you do, it just needs to be performed consistently for a period of time to make the desired changes to your body. The stark reality is that changing exercise programs too frequently does not allow your body to adapt to the work being performed, ultimately reducing the chance of experiencing the results you want.

Everyone Needs a Plan

Every type of exercise program or format works, as long as it is applied in a consistent, progressively challenging manner. For an example, let's return to *Rocky IV* and review how Rocky and Drago each prepared for their fight. Drago exercised under the supervision of Soviet sport scientists, the best in the world—more on them in a bit—who probably had a very specific program of structured intensity, while Rocky was left to train in an isolated barn and had to improvise with the limited amount of equipment available to him. The movie shows how computers, strength training machines that measured force output, and possibly drugs assisted Drago in his preparations, while Rocky did bodyweight exercises hanging off of rafters in the barn, ran hills, and used farm equipment for strength training. Of course, Rocky wins in the end, and while the movie doesn't make clear whether his edge came from his method of training or from his internal drive to avenge the death of Apollo Creed (not going to do a spoiler alert for a movie more than 30 years old), it does demonstrate that the location and equipment aren't as important as long as you have a workout plan that applies an appropriate physical challenge with each workout.

One question I'm often asked is "Is it true that changing exercises frequently to create 'muscle confusion' is the best way to get results?" The answer, overwhelmingly, is *no*! Changing exercises or types of programs too frequently or often can be ineffective because it is the progressively challenging consistency of an exercise program that causes the changes you desire. The frequent change also means that the central nervous system (CNS) does not have the opportunity to adapt to the specific exercises being performed. Compare exercise to studying a language: If you study Mandarin one month, Farsi the next month, and Spanish the following month, you won't learn any language very well. Mastering the ability to speak a language requires constant learning and refinement of proper pronunciation, tonality, and grammar skills that take a long time to develop.

Just as you have to learn the fundamentals of a language before becoming fluent, maintaining a consistent exercise program can help you experience continuous improvement that then leads to long-term results. The first step is mastering the foundational movement skills described in chapter 3; this is essential before increasing the intensity or challenge of a workout. If you change exercise programs before they have a chance to be effective, yes, you are burning calories, which is important, but you are not being consistent enough to create any significant change.

Simply put, exercise is a physical stress imposed upon the body; the actual types of exercise performed (the particular stress applied to the body) along with how often that stress is applied will determine the physical changes that happen to your body. Doing the same exercises repetitively for too long means that the various physiological systems (including muscular, metabolic, cardiorespiratory, and nervous) will adapt to the specific type of activity being performed. There are many different types of exercise stimuli, each one capable of producing a different response from the body, so it's important to have a thoughtful approach to exercise that you can apply for a sufficient amount of time to make the desired changes.

To achieve successful aging or any other fitness goal, it's important to perform a workout program consistently for 6 to 12 weeks so that the body—specifically the CNS, muscles, and metabolic pathways—can adapt to the exercise stimulus. This chapter will review the science of exercise program design so that you know which workouts to do, when to do them, and how long they should be in your program before you switch to a different type of stimulus.

Building a Foundation for Successful Aging

Every plan needs a good beginning, and exercise is no different. When it comes to exercise, long-term success is built upon the foundation of enhancing your ability to move more efficiently, which can help to reduce the risk of injury as you progress to the high-intensity exercises that are critical for successful aging. Moving more efficiently requires improving the mobility of the mobile joints, specifically the ankles, hips, intervertebral segments of the thoracic spine, and shoulders, while enhancing the stability of the stable joints, specifically the intervertebral segments of the lumbar spine, the scapulothoracic joints, the knees, and other joints structurally designed to create a platform of stability allowing you to function more efficiently. Bodyweight movements based on the patterns of hip hinge, squat, lunge, push, pull, and rotation combine joint stability with mobility to improve overall movement skill and coordination. Lower-intensity, bodyweight exercises like the glute bridge, reverse lunge, front plank, and side plank can help you to achieve or restore optimal joint function. Adding low- to moderate-intensity resistance with equipment like light dumbbells, medicine balls, and resistance cables (or tubing) can help you to develop the strength endurance to sustain muscle contractions for longer periods before you progress to the higher loads and more explosive movements that can promote muscle growth.

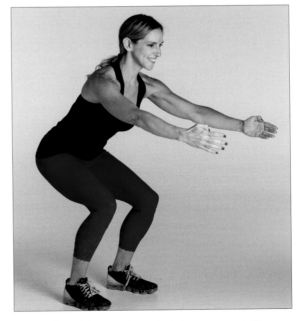

The bodyweight squat can help improve mobility of the mobile joints while enhancing stability of the stable joints.

As described in chapter 5, strength training using external resistance can improve muscle force production, eventually allowing you to lift the heavier weights responsible for stimulating the production of muscle-building hormones. Power exercises focus on speed, or the velocity of force production; therefore, the weight doesn't need to be heavy to produce the desired results. Whether it's heavier resistance to improve strength or explosive movement to increase power, repeated applications of exercise stress cause physiological adaptations so the body can become more effective at handling and overcoming these stresses. One of the foundational principles of exercise, the specific adaptations to imposed demands (SAID) principle, states that the body adapts to the specific physiological demands imposed by the exercise program. The other two basic principles of exercise program design—progression and overload—dictate that in order for exercise to be effective, it needs to challenge the body to work harder by gradually increasing the intensity of the applied stimulus (Haff and Triplett 2016). Yes, high-intensity exercise can produce many benefits, but it's not possible to keep increasing the intensity of exercise. This means that structured periods of rest should be a key component of a well-designed exercise program.

Muscles need to repair and refuel after exercise, making it necessary to allow sufficient recovery time between challenging, high-intensity workouts. This doesn't mean you can't exercise every day, but it does mean that over the course of a seven-day week you probably want to have two or three high-intensity workouts, two or three moderate-intensity workouts, and one to three low-intensity workouts. There will be some weeks when you're feeling awesome and can push for three hard workouts, while during other weeks life might get in the way and you can only handle one really hard workout and a couple of moderate-intensity ones. Note that if you're going through a stressful period at work or home, it's best to lay off the high-intensity exercise because an accumulation of too much total stress can be very bad for your body. Probably the most important training day of the week is the one that is often overlooked by active people: the rest day.

Exercise Programs to Achieve Successful Aging

When metabolic and mechanical overloads are applied to the body simultaneously during a workout, it is referred to in the research literature as *concurrent training*. Concurrent training has been shown to provide overall fitness benefits and could enhance aerobic capacity but limits the effectiveness of improving muscular strength. If the goal is purely to add muscle, concurrent training may not be the best option, but if the goal is to enhance your health to achieve successful aging, it is an effective solution and the one that will be described in the rest of this chapter (Wilson et al. 2012).

There is a difference between workouts that make you sore and those that merely cause a little discomfort. Soreness can cause muscle tightness, which changes how joints move. If a joint experiences restricted motion because of muscle tightness, an injury could result. Pain means that the body is being subjected to too much physical stress, and you should stop immediately. Exercise should create discomfort; discomfort means that your body is being pushed to work at a higher capacity. This is an effective way to think about exercise: You're trying to become comfortable being physically uncomfortable. That feeling of discomfort means that your body is being pushed to new boundaries and that you are experiencing the physical changes you are striving for in your workouts.

An exercise program that applies the SAID, progression, and overload principles is the most effective method of getting results. Six to 12 weeks, or longer, is needed before an exercise program of progressively challenging training intensity can deliver lasting results. No matter what type of exercise program you do, you need to be consistent with it and progressively increase the intensity so that you can see results.

To achieve results, you should apply the variables of exercise program design—specifically exercise selection, intensity, repetitions, sets, tempo, rest interval, frequency, and recovery (table 8.1)—in a progressively challenging manner. It is well established that physical adaptations to exercise, including muscle growth and definition, depend on the application of these variables. Systematically applying and adjusting these variables is the key to long-term success for reaching all of your fitness goals, but especially for successful aging.

Table 8.1 **Variables of Exercise Program Design**

Variable	Description	Example
Exercise selection	The exercises performed during a workout. A program that favors some exercises or muscles over others could cause muscle imbalances that become a potential source of injury. For best results, exercises should be based on the six basic patterns of human movement that require many muscles to work together to generate the forces needed for movement: • Hinging patterns, in which the hips flex and extend while both feet are in contact with the ground. • Squatting patterns, in which the hips and knees flex and extend while both feet are in contact with the ground. • Lunging or single-leg patterns, in which one foot leaves and then makes contact with the ground in a pattern similar to the actions of the gait cycle. • Pushing movements, in which the hands move away from the body to the front or to an overhead position. • Pulling movements, in which the hands move toward the body from the front or from an overhead position. • Rotational movements, in which either the thoracic spine or the pelvis rotates to provide motion.	Kettlebell goblet squat Barbell deadlift Suspension trainer row One-arm overhead press with dumbbell Rear-foot elevated split squat with dumbbells
Intensity	The specific amount of weight or external resistance used for strength training. Intensity often refers to the amount of weight used with traditional equipment such as barbells, dumbbells, or machines. In general, heavier weights are used to increase strength, while lighter weights or bodyweight allow for rapid acceleration for power training. There are different ways to refer to intensity; the workouts in this book use the repetition maximum (RM) method, which means that a weight should allow a specific number of reps before causing momentary fatigue (the inability to perform another rep). Reaching fatigue is essential for improving strength and promoting muscle growth.	10RM refers to an exercise that should cause fatigue by the 10th repetition; if an 11th rep is possible, increase the weight. For optimal results, reaching fatigue a rep or two earlier is preferable to doing additional reps, especially if fatigue is *not* achieved.

(continued)

Table 8.1   **Variables of Exercise Program Design**   *(continued)*

Variable	Description	Example
Repetitions	A single, individual action of movement at a joint or series of joints that involves three phases of muscle action: muscle lengthening, a momentary pause, and muscle shortening. Repetitions and intensity have an inverse relationship; as the intensity increases, the number of repetitions able to be performed decreases. Heavier weights can induce mechanical overload in only a few repetitions, while lighter loads or bodyweight exercises can be done for a relatively high number of repetitions to create metabolic overload or to allow for explosive movements. Repetitions can also be performed for a specific amount of time. If this is the case, the goal is to perform as many reps as possible (AMRAP) in the available amount of time.	10 reps (to achieve a 10RM) or 30 sec (AMRAP in that amount of time)
Sets	The number of repetitions or length of time a specific exercise is performed before a rest interval to allow for recovery. The number of sets in each workout is based on the amount of time available and your focus (strength, power, metabolic conditioning, or mobility).	3 or 4 sets of a core strength exercise 2 to 4 sets of a power exercise 1 to 3 sets of a mobility exercise
Tempo	The speed of movement for an exercise. The time under tension (TUT), which refers to the length of time muscle fibers are under mechanical tension from a resistance training exercise, is directly related to the tempo. Along with intensity, TUT is critical for creating the desired stimulus of either mechanical or metabolic overload. A slower tempo results in longer TUT creating more mechanical overload; an explosive tempo can result in higher levels of power and rapidly deplete ATP resulting in a greater metabolic overload.	Slow to moderate tempo for a strength exercise Explosive tempo for a power exercise Fast tempo for a metabolic conditioning exercise Slow tempo for a mobility exercise
Rest interval	Time between exercise sets. A rest interval allows replenishment of adenosine triphosphate (ATP) stores in the involved muscles and recovery from neural fatigue. Proper rest intervals are essential for increasing muscular strength and optimizing metabolic conditioning.	Resting for 30 sec between exercises Resting for 90 sec after completing a circuit of different exercises
Frequency	Number of workouts or exercise sessions within a specific period such as a week or month. Too many high-intensity workouts without proper recovery in between could lead to an overtraining injury.	2 or 3 high-intensity workouts, 2 or 3 moderate-intensity workouts, and 1 to 3 low-intensity workouts a week
Recovery	The time following exercise that the body needs to repair damaged tissues and replace spent energy. The time between workouts is when your body restores the muscle glycogen used during exercise and initiates the protein synthesis to repair damaged muscles. Exercise is the application of a physical stimulus; it is the period afterward when the body actually experiences physiological changes.	For optimal recovery, do two low- to moderate-intensity workouts after a high-intensity metabolic conditioning workout before performing another challenging, high-intensity workout.

Science and Art of Exercise Program Design

Periodization is a method of organizing workouts to alternate between periods of high-, moderate-, and low-intensity exercise in order to maximize rest and recovery. The greatest benefit of periodization is that it allows for periods of structured rest or lower-intensity workouts as a means of promoting adaptations to the physically demanding stresses of higher-intensity workouts. Exercise is when the body experiences metabolic or mechanical stress; however, it's during the recovery period after the exercise that your body repairs the muscle proteins and replaces the muscle glycogen (how muscle cells store carbohydrate to be used for energy) used to fuel the workout.

Training volume is the product of intensity or the energy pathway engaged, the number of repetitions performed and sets completed in each workout, and the frequency of workouts per week. A properly periodized program adjusts training volume on a consistent basis and requires you to plan your workouts so they focus on creating metabolic overload, mechanical overload, or a combination of the two. The science of periodization is understanding how the body adapts to the imposed stresses of exercise, whereas the art is in planning and organizing the workouts so that you can achieve your desired results.

There are two types of periodization: linear and nonlinear. It is *not* necessary to make every workout in an exercise program extremely challenging. A low- to moderate-intensity workout can help promote a complete active recovery after a high-intensity strength training day. Top strength and performance coaches around the world use periodization to help elite athletes prepare for competition; if it works for people who make millions of dollars exercising for a living, why not use the same science to help you plan for successful aging?

Linear Periodization

Linear periodization is optimal for athletes preparing for a specific competition, such as a race or triathlon, or the start of a competitive sport season. Linear periodization can also be used for nonathletes preparing for an event with a specific date, such as a wedding, an anniversary (we all want to look good at our 25th or 50th reunions), or a vacation; the goal is to perform progressively challenging workouts to properly prepare and condition for the event.

When applying linear periodization, volume and intensity are inversely related; over the course of a training cycle, as the intensity of the workouts gradually increases, the volume should decrease. Linear periodization starts with a specific date for achieving peak conditioning and then works backward to organize exercise programs into shorter lengths of time based on occasional periods of off-loading or active rest for optimal adaptation. In a linear periodization program, the segments of time can be organized into short-, intermediate-, and long-term time frames.

A program to prepare for running a marathon, where the mileage gradually increases each week and

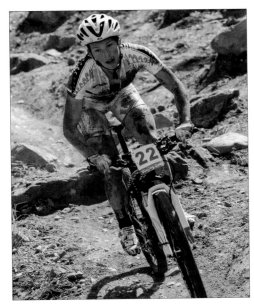

Periodization is used to help elite athletes perform at the highest levels of competition; it can help you to achieve successful aging.
Paul Gilham/Getty Images

you are supposed to take a week to 10 days of active rest before the event, is the perfect example of a linear program. Linear periodization is an extremely effective method of preparing for a date-specific event; however, since this book's purpose is to address how exercise can help you to achieve successful aging in an effort to increase your life span, assigning a specific end date is not desirable. Instead, the focus will be on applying nonlinear models so that you can learn how to stay fit and active throughout the year while reducing the risk of overtraining or developing repetitive stress injuries.

Nonlinear Periodization

The second, more practical model is nonlinear, or undulating, periodization, which adjusts the workout intensity and volume on a much more frequent basis, either from day to day or from week to week. Constantly alternating the volume and intensity of exercise can allow you to exercise every day; because some workouts will be harder while others are easier, your body will have the time to properly recover from the more intense workouts, which is essential for long-term success.

This may sound like the concept of "muscle confusion" popularized by a long-running infomercial, but that is just a marketing term. Soviet sport scientists developed the practice of undulating periodization many years ago when they realized that high-intensity workouts require longer periods of rest for optimal adaptation. As a result, they scheduled workouts that fluctuated between low, moderate, and high intensity to ensure that muscles were properly challenged while still experiencing the optimal amount of recovery time. For example, the Soviet sport scientists responsible for preparing Drago for his fight with Rocky would most likely have scheduled low-intensity training sessions the day after the hardest workouts, and about a week or so before the fight would have stopped the training altogether so that his body could fully rest, repair, and recover before the big match.

The most important component of periodization is allowing the proper rest and recovery time between hard or high-intensity workouts. As described in chapter 5, exercise applies two types of stress to your muscles: metabolic, caused by depleting the glycogen stored in individual muscle cells; and mechanical, created by physical damage to the structures of muscle proteins. Feeling sluggish or drained at the end of a workout could mean that you have indeed depleted glycogen levels, which is one purpose of a high-intensity workout; however, too many high-intensity days in a row do not provide enough time for muscles to replenish supplies of glycogen. When muscle cells don't have enough glycogen to produce ATP, the body will release the hormone cortisol, which converts protein into fuel instead of using it to repair muscle tissue. A lower-intensity workout or a day of complete rest allows your metabolism to properly replace the energy stores in your muscle cells so that you have a full supply of ATP for your next hard workout.

To allow the proper time for your body to rest, repair, and refuel, you probably want to have two or three high-intensity workouts, two or three moderate-intensity workouts, and one to three low-intensity workouts over the course of a seven-day week. You may look at that previous sentence and think, "There are only seven days in a week! How does that work?" It's necessary to acknowledge that there will be some weeks when you're feeling awesome and can crush three hard workouts, while other weeks you might be bogged down with work or other commitments and be able to handle only one really hard workout and a couple of moderate-intensity ones. The point is that the schedule should be variable so that workouts fluctuate in intensity from one day to the next.

Planning the Perfect Week of Workouts

A common misperception is that taking a day off from exercise is being lazy. Yes, it is important to be physically active most days of the week, but it is just as important to give your body a break by scheduling at least one day of complete rest about every 7 to 10 days. Even if you love to exercise and the thought of a day away from the gym or not enjoying your favorite activity makes you a little anxious, you will grow to appreciate the fact that rest is an integral component of your long-term fitness plan.

When you do make time for exercise, it might be tempting to work out as hard as possible every time you make it to the gym. But keep in mind that if you did a lot of hard, physically challenging work the day before, then your muscles may not be fully prepared to do more demanding activity. Therefore, it's important to alternate your challenging, high-intensity workouts with lower-intensity, less physically demanding but still active ones. It is a good idea to have a way to monitor the intensity of your workouts to alternate between the challenging workouts that initiate change and the lower-intensity workouts that help promote recovery from exercise.

The previously described 1 to 10 scale of the rating of perceived exertion (RPE) can be used to monitor the overall intensity of the exercise program. For best results, it is a good idea to alternate the intensity from one workout to the next. For example, if a challenging barbell strength workout at an RPE of 9/10 is done on a Monday, then the workout on Tuesday should be at an RPE of about 5 to 7/10; the lower intensity allows the body to burn calories and receive the benefits of physical activity while the tissues are going through the restoration and repair process.

Because every person is different and will have a different response to exercise, it is not possible to create a workout that will produce results for everyone. However, using the 1 to 10 scale of RPE as a guide for monitoring intensity, it can be possible to create a weekly schedule that alternates between high-, moderate-, and low-intensity workouts to ensure that when it's time to work hard, you are pushing yourself to your limits, and when it's time to let your body rest, recover, and repair, you are doing a lower-intensity workout that promotes that response (table 8.2).

Table 8.2 Weekly Nonlinear Periodization Workout Schedule—Example 1

Day	Exercise or activity	Intensity 1 to 10/10 of RPE
Sunday	Hatha yoga class	5 or 6/10 RPE
Monday	Resistance training workout	8 or 9/10 RPE
Tuesday	Hatha yoga class	5 or 6/10 RPE
Wednesday	Metabolic conditioning: Steady state	6 to 8/10 RPE
Thursday	Resistance training workout	8 or 9/10 RPE
Friday	Active rest: Long walk	3 or 4/10 RPE
Saturday	Resistance training followed by 10 min HIIT workout	8 to 10/10 RPE

Another option is to alternate between strength and power workouts; consider it a different way to design a three-day split that alternates between strength and power exercises for the resistance training workouts (table 8.3).

Day 1—Force production using external resistance, alternating between strength and power. If the first day is a strength workout, the next force workout day emphasizes power.

Day 2—Mobility workout focused on using bodyweight or light resistance

Day 3—Metabolic conditioning, which can alternate between high-intensity interval training (HIIT) and steady state based on your ability to recover between workouts and overall training schedule. For example, if you are feeling a little fatigued, then a 10-minute HIIT workout would be a better option than a 45-minute steady-state workout because you will do more work in less time, allowing more time for recovery.

Table 8.3 **Weekly Nonlinear Periodization Workout Schedule—Example 2**

Day	Exercise or activity	Intensity 1 to 10/10 RPE
Sunday	Strength workout: Dumbbell strength	7 or 8/10 RPE
Monday	Bodyweight mobility workout	4 or 5/10 RPE
Tuesday	Metabolic conditioning: Steady state (45 min)	5 to 7/10 RPE
Wednesday	Power workout: Bodyweight and kettlebells	8 or 9/10 RPE
Thursday	Mobility workout: Yoga class	5 or 6/10 RPE
Friday	Active rest: Long walk	3 or 4/10 RPE
Saturday	Metabolic conditioning: HIIT workout (<30 min total)	7 to 9/10 RPE

Benefits of Rest and Recovery

When it comes to exercise, sometimes less is more. For many people, simply making the time to exercise is a daunting challenge. But for others, taking time off of exercise for rest is an anathema to be avoided at all costs. If this is you, think again: Taking no rest days could lead to a repetitive stress injury or overtraining, which can decrease the effects of the best-designed exercise program. Probably the most important training day of the week is the one that many active people overlook: the rest day. Rest is recommended, is completely necessary to fully recover from the stresses of hard exercise, and is the best way to allow your muscles to adapt and grow after a hard workout.

Feeling stressed, feeling burned out, or having a tough time falling asleep even though you are physically exhausted is a sign of overtraining and a definite indicator that you need more recovery time after your workouts. You *need* a psychological break from exercise. Pushing through a tough workout requires mental toughness and stamina, meaning that physical exertion is hard not only on your body but on your brain as well. Spending a day away from your typical training environment can help your mind relax, allowing it to recover along with your muscles.

High-intensity exercise is like watching videos on your mobile phone: yes, you can do it, but it drains your battery quickly, meaning that you have to recharge more frequently or carry additional battery packs. High-intensity exercise causes your muscle cells to run out of stored glycogen like a phone battery after too much YouTube; it takes time to replace the expended energy. Because your body probably has an ample supply of free fatty acids that can produce ATP, you are capable of producing energy to fuel low-intensity activities below the first ventilatory threshold (VT$_1$) every day.

When your muscles have been feeling sore, a day of complete rest can allow your circulatory system to perform its job of removing the metabolic by-products in muscle cells (from using energy during exercise) while delivering the oxygen and nutrients used to repair damaged tissues. In addition, a day of complete rest allows time for the fibroblasts (individual cells that repair damaged tissues like muscle proteins) to do their job and repair any tissues damaged from the mechanical stresses of exercise. Tell yourself that you're *not* being lazy; you're focusing on the recovery phase of your workout program.

When making the transition to harder workouts or starting to exercise again after time off, do not push the intensity too quickly because trying to progress too fast could cause injury. One of the best exercises that you can perform in any week is to take time over the weekend to plan your schedule; identify and register for the classes you want to take, make plans with your friends for your workouts, or write your individual workouts into your schedule. Just as taking time to plan your meals means that you're not eating pizza for every meal, taking time to plan your workouts means that your body will get the exact physical activity it needs for each day of the week as well as optimal rest between workouts.

As you plan your workout schedule, consider what you're going to be doing before bedtime as well. A high-intensity workout requires a full night's sleep for optimal recovery, and if you have plans in the evening that include an extra drink or two or getting to sleep later than usual, then you reduce your ability to achieve optimal recovery. For example, if you have a hard workout planned for a Friday, then Friday night plans should be to watch TV and chill so that you can have a great night's sleep for your muscles. If your Friday night plans include tickets to a concert or attending a party that you know will go into the wee hours, then you're better off with a lower-intensity workout and scheduling the hard workout for another day when you will be able to get enough high-quality sleep to adequately recover.

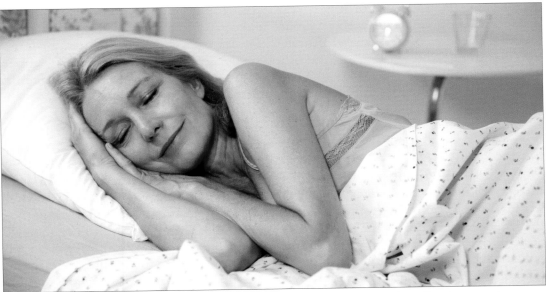

Sleep is one of the most effective methods for allowing the body to recover from the stresses of exercise. On those days that you are going to do your harder workouts, make sure that you can get a great night's sleep so your muscles can adequately recover.
BSIP/Universal Images Group via Getty Images

Here is the thing: There is no 100 percent right way to exercise, and each of us will gravitate toward the type of exercises we enjoy most. The idea is to acknowledge the role that recovery plays in your exercise program and plan your workouts accordingly so that you are performing the hardest ones on the days when you can get high-quality sleep and scheduling shorter or lower-intensity workouts on those days when you have other demands on your time or you know your rest will be compromised.

Exercise and Your Immune System

The fact that illness is the second leading cause of missing practice or playing time for athletes has given rise to a field of study known as exercise immunology; as a result, researchers have developed a good understanding about how exercise can enhance or suppress the immune system (Peake et al. 2017; Simpson et al. 2015). However, it is still too early to know exactly how exercise affects the body's ability to fight COVID-19 specifically, especially since leading scientists have noted that "there is no scientific data on how physical activity may enhance immune responses against coronaviruses" (Simpson and Katsanis 2020).

Regarding exercise's general effect on the immune system, scientists have identified a J curve showing that a certain amount of exercise may strengthen the immune system, but too much exercise at too high of an intensity with inadequate recovery time can weaken the immune system, making it more susceptible to infection (Halabchi, Ahmadinejad, and Selk-Ghaffari 2020; Gleeson 2007). As Gleeson (2007) noted, "While engaging in moderate activity may enhance immune function above sedentary levels, excessive amounts of prolonged, high-intensity exercise may impair immune function."

The human immune system has two primary subsystems: the innate immune system, which is the first line of defense against developing an infection; and the adaptive immune system, which can produce a specific response to a foreign infection. The innate immune system includes the skin, which prevents infections from entering the body; mucus membranes; acidity of bodily fluids and secretions; and leukocytes (white blood cells), which contain a number of specific cells including T cells, B cells, and natural killer (NK) cells. The adaptive immune system will produce specific antibodies and increase leukocytes to fight infections when they are introduced into the body (Hoffman 2014). In general, when a disease or infection is introduced into the body, the initial response is to increase leukocytes in an effort to eliminate the threat. The adaptive immune system can help enhance the response so that if a specific disease is reintroduced into the body, it already has the antibodies to defeat it.

The function of the first line of defense, the innate immune system, which includes the mucus linings of the nasal passages, respiratory tract, and intestines, is to keep foreign pathogens from entering the body in the first place (Simpson et al. 2015). COVID-19, like a number of diseases, is caused by an airborne virus that can enter through the body's respiratory system. Therefore, consider wearing a mask when working out or taking a group fitness class as a way to supplement and strengthen the innate immune system. Research on the use of face masks to limit the spread of airborne influenza found that "mask use not only protects healthy individuals but also reduces the infectiousness of symptomatic and asymptomatic carriers, thus reducing the number and effectiveness of transmission sources with the population. ... Mask use is virtually the only way to prevent aerosol transmission, which may cause the most severe cases of influenza. The population-wide use of face masks can be a valuable strategy to delay or contain an influenza pandemic, or at least decrease the infection attack rate" (Brienen et al. 2010).

It's important to remember that exercise is a physical stress imposed upon the body that can have both an acute and a chronic effect on the immune system. The sympathetic nervous system (SNS) and hypothalamus-pituitary-adrenal (HPA) axis are activated during exercise to promote energy metabolism; however, they also have an important impact on the immune system's ability to release the leukocytes responsible for fighting infections. In the acute phase after a single bout of moderate-intensity exercise, levels of leukocytes can increase, helping to strengthen the immune system (Simpson et al. 2015).

Overall, as Simpson and colleagues (2020) wrote, "The impact of exercise on innate and acquired immune parameters is dependent on the intensity of exercise, and in high-performance sports, the duration and load of training." The impact of exercise on the immune system is based on a number of different factors, some of which are completely variable based on the individual. Factors that regulate function of the immune system include genetics, age, nutrition, training status, underlying health conditions, psychological stress, and medical history (Simpson et al. 2020; Peake et al. 2017).

When it comes to extensive periods of high-intensity exercise or competitions, researchers have identified what they term an "open window" when the immune system is compromised, increasing the likelihood of an infection entering the body (Peake et al. 2017; Simpson et al. 2015). According to Gleeson (2007), "Various immune cell functions are temporarily impaired following acute bouts of prolonged, continuous heavy exercise and athletes engaged in intensive periods of endurance training appear to be more susceptible to minor infections." Peake and colleagues (2017) noted, "If exercise is repeated again while the immune system is still depressed, this could lead to a greater degree of immuno-depression and potentially a longer window of opportunity for infection." Simpson and colleagues (2020) observed that "arduous bouts of exercise, typically those practiced by athletes and other high-performing personnel (i.e., military), have been associated with suppressed mucosal and cellular immunity, increased symptoms of upper respiratory tract infections, latent viral reactivation and impaired immune responses to vaccine and novel antigens."

Another variable affecting exercise's impact on the immune system is the availability of glycogen and the metabolism of immune cells: "Immunometabolism is an emerging science that highlights connections between the metabolic state of immune cells and the nature of the immune response" (Simpson et al. 2020). Just like muscle cells, immune cells require fuel to function; prolonged periods of intense exercise could limit the amount of energy available for these cells and contribute to the open window phenomenon (Simpson et al. 2020). Carbohydrates ingested during and immediately after exercise could help support optimal immune function (Peake et al. 2017). Therefore, when you perform extensive periods of high-intensity activity, proper nutrition is essential for supporting optimal immune system performance.

The good news is that the research literature is in overwhelming agreement that a limited amount (less than 45 minutes) of moderate-intensity exercise can enhance the immune system and reduce the risk of becoming sick (Halabchi, Ahmadinejad, and Selk-Ghaffari 2020; Simpson et al. 2020; Peake et al. 2017; Simpson et al. 2015; Hoffman 2014; Gleeson 2007). During cold and flu season or flare-ups of COVID-19, your workouts should be of shorter duration and at low to moderate intensity to ensure that exercise is strengthening your immune system as well as the rest of your body.

Action Steps to Strengthen Your Immune System

Your exercise habits can have an important impact on strengthening your immune system to reduce the risk of developing *any* infectious disease. Based on the evidence, the following steps could help you to reduce the risk of catching COVID-19 or any other airborne disease:

- Wear a mask when exercising indoors around other individuals. Yes, it may be awkward and uncomfortable, but public health departments issued orders to wear a mask because the evidence suggests that they can help to reduce transmission. Also, consider a mask a part of your body's innate defense system against catching a disease in the first place.
- Use the scale of the rating of perceived exertion to monitor intensity; a 4 to 7/10 RPE for less than 45 minutes at a time could help to strengthen your immune system.
- Reduce the volume and duration of high-intensity exercise. When it comes to high intensity, the intensity is more important than the duration. One four-minute cycle of a Tabata protocol can be enough to improve aerobic efficiency and burn calories. Doing more than one may not provide any additional benefits and could actually weaken your immune system. At the end of the day, it simply isn't worth it.
- When possible, limit high-intensity exercise to outdoors or indoor locations with sufficient airflow where recommended distancing guidelines can be followed. High-intensity exercise increases the respiration rate, which can spread more germs; allowing for proper spacing during a workout could reduce the risk of airborne transmission.
- When you do engage in high-intensity exercise, avoid public places during the open window when the immune system is in a compromised state. "Post-exercise immune function depression is most pronounced when the exercise is continuous, prolonged (>1.5h), of moderate to high intensity (55-75% maximum O_2 uptake) and performed without food intake" (Gleeson 2007). If you work in an office around other people, avoid high-intensity exercise in the morning, which could compromise your immune system. Instead, try to schedule high-intensity workouts at the end of the day before heading home. That way, you can be safely isolated in the evening while giving your immune system time to regain its strength.
- Follow a healthy nutrition plan that includes an appropriate amount of carbohydrates. There is evidence to suggest that restricting carbohydrates could suppress the immune system (Peake et al. 2017). While weight loss and aesthetic goals may be important to you and restricting carbohydrate intake could play a role in those outcomes, during a pandemic, exercise for optimal health should take priority over appearance. "A balanced and well-diversified diet that meets the energy demands in exercising individuals is certainly a key component to maintain immune function in response to strenuous exercise" (Peake et al. 2017).
- Use proper sleep etiquette to strengthen the immune system. Sleep is when the body naturally detoxifies and repairs itself. An extra hour of sleep a night yields an additional seven hours a week, which is like sleeping for an entire extra night. A lack of sleep can increase activation of the SNS and HPA, which can further suppress the immune system. "Sleep disturbances can depress immunity, increase inflammation and promote adverse health outcomes" (Peake et al. 2017).

A Yearlong Strength and Power Workout Program to Achieve Successful Aging

Table 8.4 gives an example of a periodized plan for an entire year that alternates between strength and power training workouts to help you achieve the amount and types of resistance training recommended by the National Strength and Conditioning Association (NSCA) guidelines. The workouts follow the three-day routine described previously in the Planning the Perfect Week of Workouts section. Day 1 is force production, exercises for either strength or power; day 2 is bodyweight training to focus on mobility and core strength (this day could also include a suspension trainer workout, a yoga class, or any type of dynamic movement with little to no external resistance); and day 3 is metabolic conditioning, alternating between HIIT and steady state. In this example, the workouts are structured to help individuals who want to achieve a peak level of fitness over the summer months. The purpose is to develop a foundation of strength during cooler months and then work on high-intensity explosive exercises during summer to activate more of the muscle fibers responsible for definition and appearance. Breaking the year up into six two-month phases allows enough time (eight weeks) for adaptation to the exercise program, but changes the workouts regularly to help you to avoid becoming stuck on a plateau.

Table 8.4 **One Year Periodized Strength and Power Workout Program**

Period	Goal(s)/outcome	Examples
January–February	Barbell strength workout: This program focuses on developing a foundation of strength and muscular development. It follows the three-day rotation described previously; the force production workouts focus on strength, using a weight heavy enough to fatigue by 10 reps and then 6 reps.	4 weeks: • 10RM, 3 sets • 45 sec rest interval 4 weeks: • 6RM, 4 sets • 60 sec rest interval
March–April	Dumbbell strength workout: The first four weeks of workouts use the heavier intensity of 6RM to improve muscular development before transitioning to a higher-volume protocol of 12RM to promote muscle growth. The dumbbells allow for greater range of motion (ROM) to help improve overall strength.	4 weeks: • 6RM, 4 sets • 60 sec rest interval 4 weeks: • 12RM, 4 sets • 45 sec rest interval
May–June	Bodyweight and medicine ball power workout: The transition to explosive training will help to recruit and engage the muscle fibers responsible for definition, in addition to increasing overall energy expenditure. The first four weeks use fewer sets and longer rest intervals to allow the body to adapt to the more explosive movement speed before increasing the number of sets and shortening the rest interval to create metabolic overload.	4 weeks: • 4-6RM, 3 sets • 60 sec rest interval 4 weeks: • 5-8RM, 5 sets • 30-45 sec rest interval
July–August	Combined strength workout: This program uses dumbbells and bodyweight (via a suspension trainer) to emphasize overall strength training to maintain muscle definition and increase muscular endurance. The first four weeks is the transition back to strength training; the second four weeks increase volume while reducing rest time to create both mechanical and metabolic overload for optimal muscular development.	4 weeks: • 10RM, 3 sets • 60 sec rest interval 4 weeks: • 12RM, 5 sets • 45 sec rest interval

(continued)

Table 8.4 **One Year Periodized Strength and Power Workout Program** *(continued)*

Period	Goal(s)/outcome	Examples
September–October	Bodyweight and kettlebell power workout: This phase is a transition back to explosive training to focus on power exercises for the purpose of creating metabolic overload. The first four weeks use a lower volume for the transition back to power exercises; the second four weeks increase the number of reps and sets.	4 weeks: • 5RM, 3 sets • 45 sec rest interval 4 weeks: • 6RM, 5 sets • 45 sec rest interval
November–December	Dumbbells and suspension trainer strength workout: This time of year has many demands for time, making it difficult to schedule workouts; a strength training program using dumbbells and bodyweight (on a suspension trainer) can allow workouts to happen either at home (with the right equipment) or in a gym so that there can be no excuses for holiday weight gain. The first four weeks use four sets to transition back to strength training; the second four weeks increase the reps and shorten the rest interval to increase overall metabolic overload.	4 weeks: • 10RM, 4 sets • 60 sec rest interval 4 weeks: • 15RM, 3 sets • 45 sec rest interval

Combine Strength and Power Exercises Through Complex Training

When it's not possible to spend a lot of time in the gym, a method known as complex training can help to increase the overall power output of the muscles used in the workout. Also known as combination training, elastic equivalency training, or postactivation potentiation (PAP), complex training is a challenging system of resistance training that calls for performing two exercises for the same muscle group or movement pattern, one immediately after the other (Verkhoshansky and Siff 2009).

The first exercise uses a heavy resistance for only a few repetitions to increase motor unit activation. The second exercise focuses on explosive movement to increase the rate of force development. It's performed after a brief rest and places an emphasis on the speed of movement. The motor units are programmed by the CNS to contract; complex training helps to engage more motor units and increase the speed at which they are activated. Doing the same weights for the same reps at the same movement speed is like using an old flip phone from the early 2000s: Yes, you may be able to make calls on it, but it does not have the ability to surf the web, record videos, or use apps. Complex training improves the neural efficiency of muscle contraction, which is like upgrading to the latest iPhone capable of high-resolution digital video and looking up websites during a call.

The variables of the first exercise follow the guidelines for max strength training: an intensity of 85 to 100 percent of one-repetition max (1RM) for one to five repetitions. Then, once the max strength exercise is completed, there should be a minimal rest period, less than 30 seconds to set up for the second exercise, which uses the variables for explosive power training: an intensity of 30 to 50 percent of 1RM for four to six repetitions. The exercise of the second set should place an emphasis on accelerating all the way through an ROM such as a throw or jump. An example of complex training would be a set of heavy barbell chest presses with 90 percent of 1RM for three to five reps followed immediately by a set of bodyweight explosive hand-clap push-ups or medicine ball chest passes at 5 percent of bodyweight for four to six reps. Another example would be heavy squats for five reps followed by squat jumps for four to six reps. A third example would be heavy barbell rows for three to five reps followed immediately by straight-armed medicine ball slams for four to six reps. The rest interval would take place after the completion of both sets and would be long enough to allow for proper recovery of the energy and nervous systems, about two to four minutes.

Changing the Intensity of Your Workouts

Just because a workout feels challenging doesn't mean that it will produce the desired results. There is a major difference between a workout program that can actually produce results and one that simply feels really hard. As mentioned, overall training volume is one of the most important factors in determining the success of a workout program. Remember, volume is the amount of intensity multiplied by the number of repetitions and number of sets performed and the frequency of workouts per week. Here's a little secret: The exercises themselves are not the only way to enhance strength or improve definition. The number of sets in a workout and how they are arranged with the rest intervals can be the most important variables for achieving a specific fitness goal. The organization of the workouts can make a big difference in the overall work rate to help you to achieve the greatest benefits. Keeping the exercises consistent can help improve movement efficiency; however, to keep the muscles growing, it is necessary to apply completely new stimuli, which you can do by organizing the sets in different ways.

Exercise is a function of movement, and movement is a skill that must be developed with practice. Therefore, it *is* important to maintain consistency with the exercises you do because repetition is essential for your body to learn how to move more effectively and make the changes you want. A traditional workout design is to complete a set and rest before performing another set of the same exercise; this is called horizontal training because you complete all sets of an exercise before transitioning to a new one. This can be effective, but it is not the only way to design a workout program.

Table 8.5 provides nine different strategies for how to organize your workouts and the outcomes each method can be expected to produce. Knowing how to apply different methods of organizing workouts is especially useful if you're exercising at home with a limited amount of equipment. Simply manipulating variables such as the order in which the exercises are performed, the number of reps or sets, or the length of the rest interval can produce an entirely different workout using the same weights. In general, once an exercise feels easy, the methods for increasing the level of difficulty are to use a heavier weight, add reps, complete more sets, or reduce the rest time between sets. For best results from your workout time, follow one method for 8 to 10 weeks before switching to a new method.

Table 8.5 **Methods of Organizing Workouts**

Organizing method	Description	Example(s)
Circuit training	A series of exercises in a row featuring alternate movement patterns and body parts; exercises could be performed for a specific amount of time or a number of repetitions per station. The same exercises can be organized in a variety of different circuits so that every workout feels different, but you are staying consistent with the exercises for optimal results.	Using weights that allow 12-15 repetitions of each exercise, no rest between exercises: • Barbell deadlifts (p. 113) • Standing shoulder presses with dumbbells (p. 133) • Barbell bent-over rows with supinated grip (p. 141) • Push-ups (p. 125) • Reverse lunges with dumbbells (p. 119) • Diagonal low-to-high lifts with dumbbell (p. 148) Rest for 90 sec; repeat 3-4 times.
Sets for time	Also known as as many reps as possible (AMRAP); instead of a specific number of reps for each set, increase the workload by performing continuous reps for a specific length of time. This method creates metabolic overload while also measuring progress by counting the number of reps performed in a certain time. This allows you to push yourself without being limited by a repetition count.	• Kettlebell swings (p. 115) for 30 sec, rest for 30 sec • Push-ups (p. 125) for 30 sec, rest for 30 sec • One-arm bent-over rows with kettlebell (p. 142)—30 sec each arm, rest for 30 sec after both arms • Kettlebell clean to presses (p. 154)—30 sec each arm, rest for 30 sec after both arms

(continued)

Table 8.5 **Methods of Organizing Workouts** *(continued)*

Organizing method	Description	Example(s)
Supersets	Two exercises in a row, without any rest interval, that target opposing movements; as one muscle group is working, the other is resting, allowing you to complete more work in less time.	• Push-ups (p. 125) and dumbbell bent-over rows with supinated grip (p. 141) • Kettlebell goblet squats (p. 114) and standing shoulder presses with dumbbells (p. 133)
Compound sets	Two (or more) exercises in a row that target the same movement pattern or muscle groups to create both mechanical and metabolic overload on the involved muscles.	• Barbell deadlifts (p. 113)—Romanian deadlifts (RDLs) with barbell (p. 112)—reverse lunges with dumbbells (p. 119) • Suspension trainer push-ups (p. 126)—push-ups on ground (p. 125)—floor chest presses with dumbbells (p. 128)
As many rounds as possible	A second meaning of the acronym AMRAP; perform a circuit of exercises as many times as possible during a set time. This format will challenge you if you do not like the traditional method of resting between exercises.	A bodyweight circuit consisting of: • 15 squats • 15 push-ups • 15 reverse lunges • 15 suspension trainer rows • 15 lateral lunges Complete the circuit as many times as possible in 12 min.
Complex training (PAP) sets	Two exercises in a row for the same movement: The first exercise follows the guidelines for strength—a heavy weight for three to five repetitions; after a brief rest interval of 30 sec or less to transition to the next move, the second exercise follows the guidelines for power—explosive movement for four to six repetitions. This is an advanced exercise technique that could help create new and challenging workouts.	• Dumbbell goblet squats (p. 114) to squat jumps (p. 116) • Barbell bent-over rows with supinated grip (p. 141) to medicine ball slams (p. 144) • Push-ups (p. 125) to medicine ball chest press throws (p. 137)
Every minute on the minutes (EMOMs)	A completely different way to organize a workout: After a complete warm-up, set a timer, and at the start of every minute do a specific number of reps of an exercise. Once you are finished, you have the remainder of the minute to rest. EMOMs can either focus on one exercise like kettlebell swings or alternate between upper and lower body movements like reverse lunges with dumbbells on the even minutes and push-ups on the odd minutes.	Set a timer for 10 minutes. On the even minutes, do 20 kettlebell swings (p. 115); when you're done, rest for the remainder of the minute. On the odd minutes, do 15 push-ups (p. 125). You'll complete 5 sets of each exercise in 10 minutes.
Russian 5 × 5 method	Five sets of five reps for five different exercises. Politics aside, the former Soviet Union produced some of the best sport scientists in the world. This is one effective method they identified for improving total body strength. The goal is to use a weight heavy enough to make five reps extremely challenging. A phase of 5 × 5 training will help develop a great foundation of strength.	5 sets of 5 reps each: • Barbell deadlifts (p. 113) • Barbell bent-over rows with supinated grip (p. 141) • Incline chest presses with dumbbells (p. 127) • Romanian deadlifts (RDLs) with barbell (p. 112) • Standing shoulder presses with barbell (p. 133)
Ladder sets	Sets with increasing and then decreasing numbers of reps. These sets can add a little twist to circuit training. Select three to five exercises, and start with a low number of reps. Move from one exercise to the next with minimal rest, just long enough to switch position or grab new equipment. Each round, add more reps to "climb up" the ladder, and then reduce the number of reps to "climb down."	Sets with increasing and decreasing reps of: • Kettlebell swings (p. 115) • Push-ups (p. 125) • One-arm bent-over rows with dumbbell (p. 142) • One-arm overhead presses with dumbbell (p. 131) Complete rounds of the following for each exercise: 4 reps—6 reps—8 reps—8 reps—6 reps—4 reps To increase the level of intensity, set a timer for 8-12 minutes and try to complete the entire ladder before time runs out.

9

Extend Your Life Span

For centuries humans have sought the elusive fountain of youth, and now entire industries are built around selling billions of dollars a year of medical procedures, pills, and potions claiming to help users look years younger. Despite all of the modern efforts that have been directed toward that objective, becoming immortal like the Connor MacLeod character in *Highlander* is simply not possible. What is possible, however, is applying the latest understandings of exercise science to extend your life span by a number of years.

Biohacking is a relatively new and trendy term used to describe the process of trying to optimize the human experience through nutrition, lifestyle habits like good sleep and hygiene, and exercise. The good news is that the book you have in your hands has laid out what you need to know to use exercise to extend your life span by years of high-quality living, and all you have to do is sweat a little. As you have read, a growing body of scientific evidence strongly suggests that high-intensity exercise may provide the best pathway for retaining your youthful features while helping you to live longer. This chapter will expand on specific ways you can use exercise and physical activity to achieve better health through fitness.

Once done purely to enhance aesthetic appearance, exercise has many benefits beyond the extrinsic that can help you to change your body to improve your overall quality of life. Aging is going to happen; nothing can interrupt the progression of time. However, you can use exercise, specifically high-intensity exercise, to manage how the passage of time affects your body. From improving muscle metabolism to elevating levels of muscle-building hormones to enhancing aerobic capac-

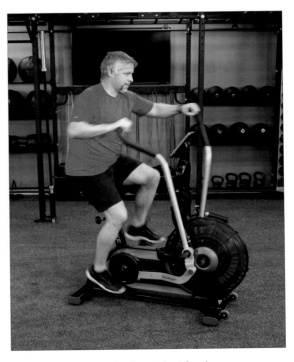

High-intensity exercise is not just for the young; as we age, it can help us to manage the effects of time on our bodies.

ity to improving cognitive function, the evidence presented in the previous chapters suggests that there are many ways high-intensity exercise can help you to preserve your youth throughout the aging process.

Where to Exercise

Now that you have learned about the many benefits of high-intensity exercise for extending your life span, it's time to identify *where* you can perform the workouts to achieve these benefits. You have many options, including working out at home, joining a health club (going forward, the term *health club* will refer to gyms and any multipurpose facilities that charge an annual membership fee, including workplace fitness centers), or going to a private studio, many of which offer only one specific modality of fitness. This section will cover how to set up a home workout space, give an overview of the rapidly growing options for streaming services that allow you to either do a prerecorded workout or follow along with a live instructor who may be leading the workout from a different time zone, and discuss how to shop for a health club or studio.

When it comes to selecting a location for your workouts, there is no one right answer. In fact, it might be best to have multiple options. Even if you pay for a monthly membership to a health club or fitness studio, it is worth your while to invest in some home equipment or a streaming service so that you can still exercise on those days when getting to a facility is not possible. There will be times when a home workout with your own equipment using either a streaming service or one of the workouts from this book will be the best option. Other times you will want the social interaction or the push to work hard that you can find at a studio or health club. The bottom line is that you want choices. As with many things in life, budget, access, and schedule will dictate the most effective solution for your needs, but don't let cost keep you from having options. Consider your investment in fitness this way: You can invest now to achieve and maintain optimal health, or you can pay for it in health care and emotional costs later when you may have to deal with a chronic disease or rapidly declining cognitive function. Making the investment now for access to exercise solutions will provide immediate benefits as well as pay dividends far into the future as you extend your life span with years of high-quality living.

Exercising at Home

Going back to the days of the Jack LaLanne television show and Jazzercise workouts on VHS tapes, exercising at home has always been a popular option. Exercising at home can be further organized into two primary categories: purchasing equipment for your own workouts or subscribing to one of many streaming services that can provide both live and previously recorded workouts led by qualified instructors. In addition, because there are so many health-conscious consumers, many housing developments now include as an amenity a full-sized, well-equipped fitness center, often with much of the same exercise equipment that can be found in commercial health clubs.

Setting up space for home workouts is not that expensive; there are many options for equipment, and the workouts provided in chapter 6 do not require much space. Streaming services range from expensive ones that require the purchase of equipment such as a mirror capable of displaying video images, a stationary bike, a treadmill, or an electronic resistance machine to cheaper ones that provide workouts requiring minimal equipment like dumbbells, elastic resistance bands, or even just your own bodyweight.

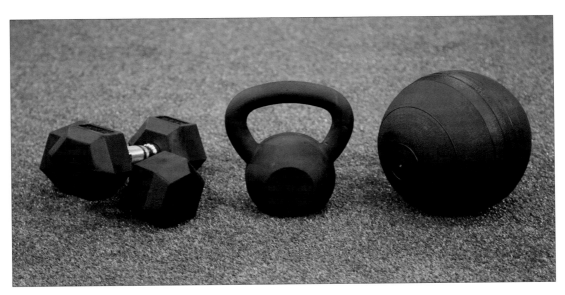

Equipment like this is very affordable and easy to store for home workouts.

Creating a Fitness Space in Your Home

Perhaps you have the motivation, budget, and space to outfit an entire fitness space at home but need to know what equipment to purchase. Keep in mind that you don't need a lot of space; often just moving the coffee table out of the way can provide more than enough space for a workout. In the best case, you may have a spare room (that's one benefit of sending a kid off to college) or a part of your garage that you can convert into a workout space.

The good news is that it is not that difficult or expensive to set up a home gym, and your budget will determine the best equipment to purchase. The following are solutions for three different budgets: less than 100 dollars (the approximate price of four studio workouts), 250 dollars (about the cost of five months of a gym membership or two months of unlimited classes at a boutique studio), and unlimited (in case your last name happens to be Gates, Bezos, or Zuckerberg). Note that professional distributors like Perform Better and Power Systems that sell commercial-grade equipment to health clubs, university conditioning programs, and professional teams are a much better option when shopping for smaller home equipment than the world's largest online book seller; the commercial-grade equipment might be a little more expensive, but it is designed and built to last longer than generic consumer pieces.

Less Than 100 Dollars

- *Stretch mat*—A good stretch mat will make ground-based mobility exercises much more comfortable.
- *Foam roller*—This is important for reducing muscle tightness and creating optimal mobility.
- *Set of dumbbells*—Many of the big box retailers that sell groceries also sell fitness equipment. Select a pair that is challenging after 8 to 10 reps; as you become stronger, just keep doing more reps until you reach fatigue.
- *Two-arm resistance band*—This band can easily be attached to a door frame and allows you to replicate a number of cable machine exercises while at home.

Approximately 250 Dollars: All of the Above Plus These

- *Relatively heavy medicine ball*—There are two types of medicine balls: those that bounce and those that don't (sometimes called slam balls). For the workouts in this book, invest in one that doesn't bounce and is approximately 5 percent of your bodyweight.

- *Kettlebell*—Many big box retailers now sell kettlebells, which can be used for the strength, power, or metabolic conditioning workouts in this book. If you're purchasing only one kettlebell, select a heavier weight for power exercises like swings or goblet squats for lower body strength. It sounds counterintuitive, but when it comes to swings, a heavier kettlebell forces you to use proper technique. Using a lighter kettlebell could allow poor form, possibly resulting in an injury.

- *Additional set of dumbbells*—This is so that you have a lighter pair for upper body exercises and a heavier pair for strengthening your lower body.

Unlimited Budget: All of the Above Plus These

- *Suspension trainer*—Purchase a commercial version for an extremely versatile piece of long-lasting equipment; I recommend TRX suspension trainers. This book describes several suspension trainer exercises, and TRX makes a wide variety of exercises available online or through their app; they provide many resources for how to use their products. The TRX was developed by a Navy SEAL and has become a standard piece of fitness equipment in high-performance conditioning centers around the world. Search on YouTube to see an interview and workout I did with Randy Hetrick, the creator; I'm a big fan of the product because it's perfect for home workouts and it delivers results!

- *Second, heavier kettlebell*—Heck, if you can afford it, get a whole rack of dumbbells and three or four kettlebells to have the widest variety of exercise options.

- *Olympic weight bar and about 200 pounds of Olympic-sized weights*—This is the perfect option for a garage workout space or a basement-type workout room; investing in a bar and weights will allow you to do heavier lifts like deadlifts, bent-over rows, and Romanian deadlifts without having to go to a gym. If your budget (and space) allows, you will also want to purchase a squat rack and an adjustable bench, but a bar and weights are essential if you have the space and can afford them.

- *A high-intensity interval training (HIIT) bike or indoor rower*—Using both the upper and lower body at the same time during aerobic activity can increase the number of calories you burn. Perform an Internet search for companies that sell used commercial gym equipment; again, this could be more expensive, but commercial-grade equipment is built to higher standards and is much higher quality than the products sold via normal retail channels like sporting goods stores. Plus, investing in good equipment will motivate you to use it more often, while trying to save a few bucks to buy a consumer product that isn't well built (or that you have to assemble yourself) may leave you frustrated in the long run. Finally, a high-quality piece of used commercial equipment will have some resale value; the same cannot be said for products purchased at a sporting goods store. Note that I don't suggest buying a treadmill because you can walk or run outside. Plus, HIIT bikes and rowers are ergometers, which, as described in chapter 7, have the ability to measure the amount of work performed; however, what makes them great for home use is that the more effort you use, the more resistance is applied against you without having to make any adjustment to settings. This makes them perfect for the HIIT intervals recommended in chapter 7 because as you increase your speed of movement, the resistance automatically increases and elevates your overall work effort.

Home Workout Streaming Services

Many of the top fitness brands and studio chains are now offering some type of exercise-at-home streaming service. Some offer workouts that are prerecorded, and you can select from a wide variety of options. Others offer live classes in real time. Most of the streaming services offer mobility, strength training, and HIIT workouts that can help you to achieve the benefits described in this book. However, if you decide to go this route, make sure you do your research to ensure that the instructors have the proper qualifications to be leading the workouts and that you have the right equipment for the workouts. At the bare minimum, a fitness instructor, whether virtual or in real life, should have either a college degree in the field of exercise science or a professional certification from an accredited agency like the American Council on Exercise (ACE), the National Academy of Sports Medicine (NASM), the Athletics and Fitness Association of America (AFAA), or the American College of Sports Medicine (ACSM). A professional credential like a certification ensures that an instructor has the baseline knowledge to develop and lead exercise programs for healthy adults.

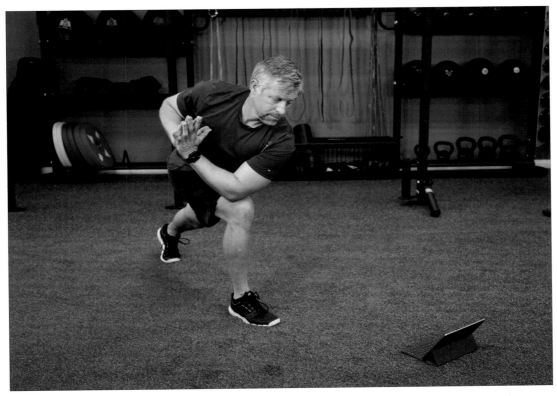

Streaming and recorded workouts that can be delivered to any device have become extremely popular and can be a convenient way to do your high-intensity exercise.

Streaming Services for Home Workouts

Already popular before the spring of 2020, video streaming services that offer workouts directly to your favorite device anywhere you have a high-speed Internet connection experienced explosive growth during the COVID-19 pandemic. Even if you pay for a health club membership, a streaming service might be worth the investment so that you have options on those days your schedule simply won't allow you to make it to a facility. A streaming service can go with you when you hit the road, so that you can still access workouts that you are familiar with and enjoy when your travel schedule takes you out of your routine.

The following are services that offer streaming workouts. Some are affiliated with national brands, and some may require investing in specific equipment; all have qualified instructors who are skilled in teaching in this medium. This is by no means an exhaustive list, and many fitness instructors offer their own workout options via videoconferencing platforms. Those listed offer a variety of programming options at different price points so that you can search for the one that best suits you. Do your research to find the best solution for your needs and budget.

Peloton

One of the early adopters of video streaming group workouts, Peloton originally offered only indoor cycling classes but has expanded to offer both live and recorded workouts for their treadmill as well. It's important to point out that while the company sells treadmills and indoor bikes under their brand name, any bike or treadmill can be used for their workouts, the primary difference being in how the equipment is adjusted for intensity. In addition, the Peloton app offers a variety of exercise formats including stretch, meditation, and strength training that do not require investing in expensive exercise equipment. You can join the service for indoor cycling or treadmill workouts or subscribe to their app as a digital member for access to the other content. One unique feature of Peloton is the group chats that allow class participants to interact with each other and the instructor, which delivers some of the benefits of a boutique studio experience wherever you can stream a workout.

The Mirror

This is one of the cleverest products on the market; rather than being a piece of specialized fitness equipment like a bike or treadmill that could end up becoming an expensive clothes hanger, The Mirror is a functional mirror that can hang on the wall, allowing you to use it for that purpose. But The Mirror is also a video monitor that connects to Wi-Fi and displays on its surface a hologram of an instructor leading a workout. You follow along to the image of the instructor, watching your reflection and matching your movements to those of the instructor to ensure that you are using the proper form and correct technique for each exercise. There is a cost for The Mirror unit itself as well as the monthly programming fee, which includes workouts ranging from strength training to HIIT to yoga and meditation. You can enjoy the fun and engaging workouts while you literally watch yourself move into better shape.

LES MILLS On Demand

LES MILLS is one of the leading group fitness class programs in health clubs all over the world and now offers a wide variety of programming, including HIIT, cardio, and strength training workouts, through its LES MILLS On Demand streaming service. LES MILLS researches its exercise formats to develop the right programming for different fitness levels and invests a lot of resources in training its instructors to be dynamic and engaging. With more than 1,000 prerecorded workouts and new ones added every month, the streaming service offers classes from 15 to 50 minutes in length. LES MILLS On Demand instructors are so engaging and dynamic that even though you may be taking a recorded class, you will feel like each one is speaking directly to you throughout the workout.

Kira Stokes Fit App

Created by celebrity fitness instructor and industry veteran Kira Stokes, this app features the Stoked Method, Kira's unique brand of fitness that combines strength training, mobility, and HIIT into the same workout. Although there are a variety of workout programs and challenges to follow, the app allows you to create fitness on your own terms by mixing and matching workouts to create the perfect program for your needs. All workouts are fully guided by Kira, who does every exercise with you while providing precise, easy-to-follow form cues and instructions. Full disclosure: Kira is an old friend; we worked together for years. I would not recommend her programming if I didn't hold her in such high regard. She truly is one of the best in the business.

Apple Fitness+

Apple Fitness+ provides workouts on demand from some of the leading instructors in the fitness industry and features all types of modalities, from treadmill running to HIIT to strength training and even indoor rowing. Because it's Apple, Fitness+ can be accessed from Apple devices such as iPhone, iPad, and Apple TV. During the session, the metrics from your Apple Watch are shown on the screen and come to life for moments of inspiration. Not only can you select workouts based on format, intensity, or length, but with Apple Music integration, you can select your fitness experience based on the music, making it perfect if you rely on tunes to push you through a challenging workout.

TRX On Demand and TRX App

The TRX suspension trainer is a versatile piece of fitness equipment that provides great workouts for strength and metabolic conditioning at home. Without a formal education in exercise science, it is not the most intuitive fitness product to learn how to use, but never fear! The team at TRX has created TRX On Demand to provide users with an extensive variety of video workouts available on their website (trxtraining.com). In addition, the company has a robust TRX app available for mobile devices; with a set of TRX straps and the app, you can get a great workout almost anywhere.

Health Club or Fitness Studio?

The first and most important point to consider when evaluating health clubs and fitness studios is the type of fitness experience that will best suit your needs. Do you want to join a health club that offers a variety of equipment, fitness classes, and amenities like a full-service locker room, or take classes from a fitness studio that might have dynamic and fun classes but doesn't offer equipment that you can use on your own or even provide a locker room with showers? There is no right or wrong answer to this question; you simply need to decide what type of fitness experience will meet your needs and, of course, budget. Some boutique studios offer only one fitness format, like indoor cycling, yoga, barre, high-intensity circuit training, or Pilates; they may charge either a fee per class, where you make reservations and pay through a mobile app (this makes them convenient for people who enjoy different fitness experiences from day to day), or monthly membership fees like a health club. Studios may offer unique programming that you can't find at other places, but many have only a changing room with no showers, so you have to plan around that reality. Plus, studios often charge a monthly fee that may be higher than that at a health club, and while they offer great classes, you don't have the option to come in and use the equipment on your own. As you consider your options, give attention to the following factors.

Convenience

Is the location convenient for you? Is it close to your home or office? This is critical because if it is out of your way, you may find excuses not to go, but if you drive past it every day or can easily bike or walk to it, there are no excuses not to go. The best option is a facility close to where you live or work so that you can easily make it a part of your daily routine. It doesn't matter how nice a facility is or how great the instructors are if it's not convenient to get to.

If you drive to the facility, does it offer convenient parking? The location may be easy to get to, but if you can't find parking when you're there or if you have to pay extra, that creates a barrier.

Formats Offered

Do you want to join a studio that focuses on only one format of exercise, or do you want access to a variety of class formats? Even if a studio only offers a single format like indoor cycling or interval training, they should be scheduling different workouts on different days. For example, one day might focus on HIIT exercise while another day features endurance training. Most health clubs have group fitness studios that offer a wide variety of programming options, meaning that you might be able to take a yoga class one day and a strength training workout the next day.

Equipment Usage

Do you want the freedom to use exercise equipment on your own? Having access to equipment means that you can follow the exercise programs in this book or do your favorite exercises on your own.

Price

How much do you want to spend per month? A number of health clubs offer month-to-month memberships that can be cancelled with 30 days' notice. But these can be significantly more expensive than a membership that has an annual contract. Here's a little secret: A club can only claim the revenue for the contracts on hand, so the more yearlong membership contracts it sells, the greater the amount of revenue on the books. Therefore, it's in a facility's best interest to have members on an annual contract since month-to-month members provide only 30 days of membership revenue. A health club with monthly dues of 50 dollars and up might seem expensive, but compare that to fitness studios that often charge 20 dollars and up per class, which can get expensive rather quickly. It's important to know that most studios strictly enforce a 24-hour cancellation policy, so if you make a reservation and pay for a Wednesday class on a Monday but get stuck working late, you are also stuck paying for a class that you can't attend.

A majority of studios that offer a specific format of exercise like barre, indoor cycling, or instructor-led, high-intensity circuit training workouts charge 150 dollars and up per month. The upside is that you receive an unlimited number of classes led by an instructor trained in how to deliver that specific format. While the price point might seem expensive, the fact that you receive customized group workouts under the supervision of a trained instructor and can attend as many workouts as you want in a month means that the more often you go, the less you pay per visit. An additional benefit is that if you attend workouts at a consistent time, you usually work out with the same people, leading to new friendships, expanding your real-life social networks, and helping you to stay committed to your goals. If you're intimidated to try high-intensity exercise on your own but want the benefits described in previous chapters, then a studio featuring instructor-led, high-intensity circuit training might work well for you.

Personal training studios are another option allowing you to work with a certified personal trainer one-on-one or in a small group, which can be an excellent way to get the instruction and guidance you need to achieve the life-promoting benefits of exercise. This can work well if you want the accountability, guidance, and structure of personalized workouts. The challenge is that this personalized service is expensive: personal training sessions can cost 50 dollars per hour and up. Some studios charge a monthly fee based on the number of sessions you attend per month and allow you to work with a variety of different trainers, which may enhance the experience.

Other Considerations

If you live in a climate that makes exercising outdoors possible most of the year, consider a bootcamp-style fitness class. Before you join one of these outdoor classes, check with your local park service or city administrator to verify that the instructor has the appropriate permission to hold a class in public. Many jurisdictions require fitness instructors to pay a fee to conduct outdoor workouts on public property. If the class doesn't have a permit, then the best worst-case scenario could involve an official showing up to escort you and the others off the property and you losing your investment in the class. The worst worst-case scenario would be that the instructor does not have liability insurance to cover accidents. If an instructor does have the appropriate permits, they likely have the necessary insurance to compensate participants in the event that any of them are injured during the workout. Given the level of difficulty of many bootcamp-style workouts, this is an extremely important consideration.

Fitness studios provide a wide variety of exercise options that have not traditionally been offered by commercial health clubs. If you are considering going to a studio because you enjoy group workouts, consider these facts about health clubs.

- Many commercial health clubs offer a number of scheduled classes that are included in the cost of the monthly membership, and they provide a wide variety of equipment such as treadmills, elliptical trainers, resistance training machines, and free weights, so you have lots of choices to meet your fitness needs.

- They may have perks such as locker rooms with amenities like towel service, saunas, whirlpools, and snack bars that are simply not available at most studios.

- Health clubs offer personal training sessions, and most hire only qualified, certified personal trainers, so you can be sure that you're working with someone who can help you reach your goals.

- Health clubs may offer fee-based, small-group training programs, which can create a studio experience.

- If you have a favorite instructor at a boutique fitness studio, search the group fitness schedules at the health clubs in your area; most instructors teach at more than one location and will often teach a couple of classes at a club in order to get a free membership.

Only you can decide which facility will meet your needs. For example, if you enjoy a specific type of programming, then by all means go the studio route. However, if you want the most options for your dollar, then a health club might offer the greatest return on investment. As you shop around, be honest with yourself about what you can afford and what you want to receive for your money.

Shopping for a Fitness Studio or Health Club

As someone who has spent more than 10 years in club operations (from front desk to general manager to national director) and another 10-plus years consulting with health clubs to educate and certify personal trainers, I can offer some unique insights to help you choose an option that is right for your needs.

First, determine your budget. Don't be tempted to overspend on a "luxury" fitness experience or a series of instructor-led workouts, especially if you're putting the expense on a credit or debit card each month (the way most clubs and studios require that you pay for membership or ongoing classes). Identify what you can realistically afford based on your personal budget, and use that to help guide your decision-making process.

You get what you pay for. If you join a gym simply because it is the lowest-priced option, then you will often have to pay extra for amenities like group classes or even towels. Low-cost gyms operate on extremely thin margins, so if equipment breaks, it can take time to repair. Staff is frequently overworked and underpaid, resulting in a lot of turnover. When visiting a health club, especially one that offers low membership fees, ask the salesperson how long they have worked there and how long the managers (general manager, fitness manager, and operations manager) have been in place. If the answers are "I don't know" or "less than six months," then the location might experience frequent staff turnover, which can have a significant effect on your membership experience.

Ask for a trial membership. You could also see if you can do a series of beginner classes before making a long-term commitment to a club or studio. Most facilities know that the best way to sell themselves is to simply let people use them, offering a reduced price for a series of beginner classes, a free trial membership for a week, or even a monthly pass so you can see if the facility meets your needs. A club or studio may charge for an initial pass because they need to cover their costs (many are franchises owned by an individual, and they need to generate a positive cash flow) but then apply that charge to the membership fee if you join in the first 30 days. Take advantage of these monthly passes to see if you like the instructors and the techniques they teach. If you don't feel comfortable doing the exercises after the initial visits, then you will probably not enjoy the long-term exercise experience. If you do a trial membership at a health club, visit during the hours you would regularly attend so that you can see how crowded it is, and try a couple of group fitness classes to see if you like the formats and instructors.

Cleanliness counts. When visiting a facility or doing a trial workout, look closely at the equipment, both underneath and on top, and in the corners for any significant collections of dust. A well-maintained facility will be clean and relatively dust-free; if you see an accumulation of dust or dirt on equipment, then that could also mean an accumulation of disease-causing germs. Another thing to pay attention to is the locker room or changing area. If it has a damp, musty, or mildewy smell, then regular cleaning is not a high priority for the facility, and nothing can ruin your fitness experience faster than having to change or try to get clean in a dirty locker room.

Look into discounts or reimbursements. Check with your employer or health insurance to see if they offer any discounts or reimbursements for health club dues or fitness facility fees. Because the Affordable Care Act makes prevention a priority, both private employers and health insurance companies have been given more leeway on the financial incentives they can provide for fitness, which is one of the best forms of prevention. Many health clubs will offer a discounted membership fee if you belong to a specific health insurance plan, but they will never tell you this during a tour, and you may have to tell them that you qualify for the discount. If your employer has an education reimbursement, they may allow you to use it to pay for a fitness class. When I was personal training full time, I wrote a couple of letters for clients stating that I was providing "fitness education services" so that they could use their company education funds to pay my fees.

Read reviews. Use the Internet to see how customers and members rate their experience at a health club or studio. Doing a search on Google or Yelp or simply asking your Facebook network about their experience with a fitness provider can deliver a wealth of information to help you to make an informed decision. Check the facility's website and social media channels to see what type of information they push out to their members. Many of the larger clubs have blogs, articles, or videos to educate members on exercise, nutrition, and lifestyle strategies that can be extremely useful and relevant for achieving fitness goals.

Check credentials. Before you make a commitment and invest your hard-earned money in a club, make sure their instructors have the appropriate professional credentials—specifically a proper, accredited certification. Here is a startling fact: The fitness industry is self-regulating, and people can call themselves personal trainers or teach an exercise class without going through any formal education or licensing process.

Timing is important. Health clubs and studios have monthly sales and membership goals and will offer special pricing in the last few days of the month to make sure they meet these goals. Waiting until the end of a month to shop for a club or studio might mean a better price or, at the very least, an additional month of membership at no additional cost.

Be an educated consumer. Think of a gym membership as an investment in your health, well-being, and longevity: It might seem expensive, but if it means that you avoid a chronic health condition while adding years to your life, it will certainly be worth it. Set your budget, do your homework, and visit the facility a few times before making a long-term financial commitment. Choosing a health club is a lot like finding a significant other: It may take a while to find the right one, but once you do, it will significantly enhance your quality of life. If a facility feels right, go for it. You'll enjoy the opportunity to exercise and meet new people. If a facility doesn't feel right, is not able to answer your questions, is too expensive (or too cheap), or is simply dirty, skip it and keep looking for the right one. You'll find it, and once you do, you'll be glad you made the extra effort.

Keep Moving Throughout Your Day

High-intensity exercise may be an essential component of successful aging, but exercise is not the only form of physical activity that can help promote health benefits. The human body burns approximately five calories of energy to consume one liter of oxygen. Because high-intensity exercise can involve a lot of muscle mass, it can definitely be effective at burning calories. In addition to structured exercise bouts, it's important to remain active throughout your day, especially if one of your exercise goals is to manage a healthy bodyweight. Even small amounts of physical activity can deliver benefits. While high-intensity exercise can increase muscle-building hormones as well as elevate levels of brain-boosting brain-derived neurotrophic factor (BDNF), consistent activity throughout the day is essential for achieving optimal health.

Remember that nonexercise activity thermogenesis (NEAT), introduced in chapter 7, can help you to burn calories throughout your day. Exercise is a physical activity performed for a specific purpose, while NEAT is the physical activity you perform throughout the course of your day, such as taking the stairs, walking for an errand (instead of driving), or doing chores around the house. It could add up to an additional 300 calories of energy expenditure per day. Increasing daily NEAT by 200 calories (the equivalent of walking about 2 miles) while making healthier nutritional choices to reduce caloric intake by 300 calories (the equivalent of a 12-ounce soda and a small bag of potato chips) equals about 500 calories a day. A pound of body fat can provide approximately 3,500 calories worth of energy; this means that by making those small changes over the course of seven days, you could reach the amount of calories necessary to eliminate a pound of fat. Through NEAT, adding seemingly small amounts of physical activity to your daily habits on top of the workouts you'll do in the gym can allow you to manage a healthy bodyweight, which is critical for optimal health throughout the aging process.

The following suggestions can add more opportunities to move throughout the day.

Make physical activity part of your daily commute to work. This may not be possible in all communities, although a number of state and local governments have added bike lanes and multiuse trails in an effort to promote cycling and walking as viable modes of transportation. While running, walking, or cycling to work may take a little longer and require some planning, the benefit is that you burn calories while those stuck in traffic are burning dollars in the form of wasted gasoline. An electric bike with a small motor to help with the hills could give you the benefit of being more active without arriving at work dripping in sweat.

Make your errands active. Perform your errands by walking or cycling. Think about the errands you run and the stores you visit on a regular basis. How many of them are within two or three miles of your home? An overlooked benefit of riding a bike to the grocery store is that it can help eliminate unnecessary purchases because you have only a limited amount of space in a backpack or saddlebag to carry what you bought. Make a trip to the store a family affair by bringing your kids or grandkids along. This sets a positive example about being more active and can also provide benefits such as physical activity for them, additional family time for everyone, and mini-Sherpas to help you carry purchases back home.

Stand more. Standing uses more muscles than sitting. Using a standing desk at work or making time for frequent standing breaks throughout your day can pay big dividends in terms of burning additional calories. As more companies understand the negative health consequences of sitting for too long, they are investing in standing desks and allowing employees opportunities to be more active throughout the day. If using a standing desk is not possible, consider performing tasks like making a phone call, typing a text, or checking your email on a mobile device while standing. Instead of buying your morning java at a shop close to your home or office, walk to another coffee shop a block or two away. Invite a couple of colleagues along to have a work-related conversation during the trip, making it productive and efficient!

Take the stairs. As more organizations try to stem health care costs by promoting physical activity at work, they are beginning to allow employees to use stairs once reserved for emergencies. If you find that you are wasting time waiting for an elevator to go visit a colleague only one or two floors away, ask your office or building manager if it is possible to have access to the stairs. You can also use the stairs in apartment buildings, parking garages, health care facilities, hotels, and shopping centers.

Park farther away. When you drive somewhere, park farther away from your destination than you normally do to give yourself the opportunity to get in extra steps. Consider that when driving to the closest parking spots you have to navigate other cars looking for close spots or shoppers strolling with no sense of urgency while carrying their purchases out of the store. Parking far from the entrance of a store serves two benefits: one, you get more activity by walking across the parking lot to your destination, and two, it is easier to drive away when you are parked closer to the exit, which is a bonus when the stores are busy.

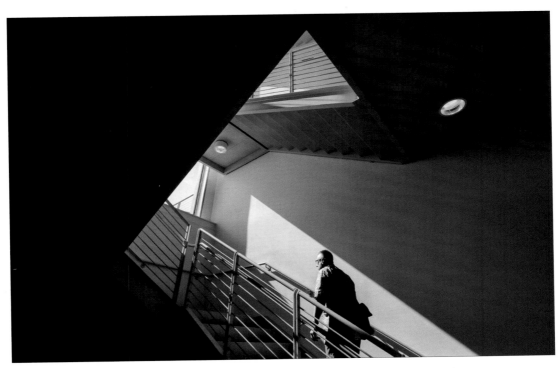

Taking the stairs can be a convenient way to keep burning calories throughout your day.
Gary Hershorn/Getty Images

Play. Enjoy time playing with your kids or grandkids. I can't tell you how many times I go to a park and see parents sitting on a bench hunched over their phones while their kids are breaking a sweat on the playground. In this modern era of an app for everything, there is no app (nor should there be) for spending time with loved ones. If you can carve out even a few minutes for playing catch, kicking a ball, or walking down to your neighborhood park, you will be spending precious time with your offspring while racking up NEAT. An additional benefit to playing is that it can actually help boost neural activity and cognition, so you increase your brain function while having fun.

Advice From a Great Philosopher

Chronological aging is inevitable. Until a real-life Doc Brown invents the flux capacitor to make time travel possible, there is nothing that can be done to arrest the forward progress of time. This leaves you with two choices: You can let life happen to you and wake up one day realizing that you are out of shape, are in poor health, and have to pay hundreds of dollars per month to manage an otherwise preventable health condition like obesity; or you can take control of your life by being active every day and doing high-intensity exercise at least two days per week so that your biological age becomes younger than your chronological age.

Here's the thing: If you are fit and healthy, then you have choices for how you can live your life. Fitness is having the ability to do what you want to do when you want to do it. A shorter way to say this is that fitness is freedom; if you are fit, you are free to go out and live your life to the fullest. If you are fit, you can take the vacations you want, you can enjoy your favorite activities well into your later years, you can discover new activities that bring joy to your life, you can keep up with your kids or grandkids, and you *will* add years of quality living to your life span. As the renowned 1980s philosopher Ferris Bueller once said, "Life moves pretty fast. If you don't stop and look around once in a while, you could miss it." Now put down this book, go lift something heavy, move until you are sweaty and out of breath, and start taking control of how the passage of time affects you so that you can live your life to its fullest potential.

References

Chapter 1

Bet da Rosa Orssatto, L., E. Cadore, L. Andersen, and F. Diefenthaeler. 2019. "Why Fast Velocity Resistance Training Should Be Prioritized for Elderly People." *Strength and Conditioning Journal* 41 (1): 105-14.

Cook, G. 2010. *Movement*. Santa Cruz, CA: On Target.

Fragala, M., E. Cadore, S. Dorgo, M. Izquierdo, W. Kraemer, M. Peterson, and E. Ryan. 2019. "Resistance Training for Older Adults: Position Statement From the National Strength and Conditioning Association." *Journal of Strength and Conditioning Research* 33 (8): 2019-52.

Katula, J., W. Rejeski, and A. Marsh. 2008. "Enhancing Quality of Life in Older Adults: A Comparison of Muscular Strength and Power Training." *Health and Quality of Life Outcomes* 6 (45): 1-8.

Physical Activity Council. 2019. *2019 Physical Activity Council Participation Report*. Jupiter, FL: Sports Marketing Surveys.

Starrett, K. 2015. *Becoming a Supple Leopard*. Las Vegas: Victory Belt.

Tabata, I., K. Irisawa, M. Kouzaki, K. Nishimura, F. Ogita, and M. Myachi. 1997. "Metabolic Profile of High Intensity Intermittent Exercises." *Medicine & Science in Sports & Exercise* 29 (3): 390-95.

Volaklis, K., M. Halle, and C. Meisinger. 2015. "Muscular Strength as a Strong Predictor of Mortality: A Narrative Review." *European Journal of Internal Medicine* 26 (15): 303-10.

Zatsiorsky, V., W. Kraemer, and A. Fry. 2021. *Science and Practice of Strength Training*. 3rd ed. Champaign, IL: Human Kinetics.

Chapter 2

Alzheimer's Association. 2019. "Alzheimer's Disease Facts and Figures." *Alzheimer's & Dementia* 15 (3): 321-87.

Baker, J., M. Bemben, M. Anderson, and D. Bemben. 2006. "Effects of Age on Testosterone Responses to Resistance Exercise and Musculoskeletal Variables in Men." *Journal of Strength and Conditioning Research* 20 (4): 874-81.

Benedict, C., S. Brooks, J. Kullberg, R. Nordenskjold, J. Burgos, M. Le Greves, L. Kilander, et al. 2013. "Association Between Physical Activity and Brain Health in Older Adults." *Neurobiology of Aging* 34:83-90.

Bet da Rosa Orssatto, L., E. Cadore, L. Andersen, and F. Diefenthaeler. 2019. "Why Fast Velocity Resistance Training Should Be Prioritized for Elderly People." *Strength and Conditioning Journal* 41 (1): 105-14.

Byrne, C. 2016. "Ageing, Muscle Power and Physical Function: A Systematic Review and Implications for Pragmatic Training Interventions." *Sports Medicine* 46 (9): 1311-32.

Candow, D., P. Chilibeck, S. Abeysekara, and G. Zello. 2011. "Short-Term Heavy Resistance Training Eliminates Age-Related Deficits in Muscle Mass and Strength in Older Males." *Journal of Strength and Conditioning Research* 25 (2): 326-33.

Chaddock, L., M. Voss, and A. Kramer. 2012. "Physical Activity and Fitness Effects on Cognition and Brain Health in Children and Older Adults." *Kinesiology Review* 12 (1): 37-45.

Chang, Y., and J. Etnier. 2009. "Exploring the Dose-Response Relationship Between Resistance Exercise Intensity and Cognitive Function." *Journal of Sport and Exercise Psychology* 31 (5): 640-56.

Chang, Y., C. Pan, F. Chen, C. Tsai, and C. Huang. 2012. "Effect of Resistance-Exercise Training on Cognitive Function in Healthy Older Adults: A Review." *Journal of Aging and Physical Activity* 20:497-517.

Church, D., J. Hoffman, G. Mangine, A. Jajtner, J. Townsend, K. Beyer, R. Wang, et al. 2016. "Comparison of High-Intensity vs. High-Volume Resistance Training on the BDNF Response to Exercise." *Journal of Applied Physiology* 121:123-28.

Ciolac, E., G. Brech, and J. Greve. 2010. "Age Does Not Affect Exercise Intensity Progression Among Women." *Journal of Strength and Conditioning Research* 24 (11): 3023-30.

Fragala, M., E. Cadore, S. Dorgo, M. Izquierdo, W. Kraemer, M. Peterson, and E. Ryan. 2019. "Resistance Training for Older Adults: Position Statement From the National Strength and Conditioning Association." *Journal of Strength and Conditioning Research* 33 (8): 2019-52.

Godfrey, R., and A. Blazevich. 2004. "Exercise and Growth Hormone in the Aging Individual, with Special Reference to the Exercise-Induced Growth Hormone Response." *International SportMed Journal* 5 (4): 246-60.

Goto, K., N. Ishii, T. Kizuka, and K. Takamatsu. 2005. "The Impact of Metabolic Stress on Hormonal Responses and Muscular Adaptations." *Medicine and Science in Sports and Exercise* 37 (6): 955-63.

Gries, K., U. Raue, R. Perkins, K. Lavin, B. Overstreet, L. D'Acquisto, B. Graham, et al. 2018. "Cardiovascular and Skeletal Muscle Health with Lifelong Exercise." *Journal of Applied Physiology* 125:1636-45.

Haff, G., and N. Triplett. 2016. *Essentials of Strength and Conditioning*. 4th ed. Champaign, IL: Human Kinetics.

Häkkinen, K. 2011. "The Aging Neuromuscular System in Men and Women Still Responds to Strength Training." Lecture given at the NSCA National Conference, Las Vegas, NV, July 6-9, 2011.

Izquierdo, M., K. Häkkinen, J. Ibanez, M. Garrues, A. Anton, A. Zuniga, and J.L. Larrion. 2001. "Effects of Strength Training on Muscle Power and Serum Hormones in Middle-Aged and Older Men." *Journal of Applied Physiology* 90:1497-507.

Jimenez-Maldonado, A., I. Renteria, P. Garcia-Suarez, J. Moncada-Jimenez, and L.F. Freire-Royes. 2018. "The Impact of High-Intensity Interval Training on Brain-Derived Neurotrophic Factor in Brain: A Mini-Review." *Frontiers in Neuroscience* 12:839.

Katula, J., W. Rejeski, and A. Marsh. 2008. "Enhancing Quality of Life in Older Adults: A Comparison of Muscular Strength and Power Training." *Health and Quality of Life Outcomes* 6 (1): 45-53.

Kersick, C., C. Wilborn, B. Campbell, M. Roberts, C. Rasmussen, M. Greenwood, and R. Kreider. 2009. "Early-Phase Adaptations to a Split-Body, Linear Periodization Resistance Training Program in College-Aged and Middle-Aged Men." *Journal of Strength and Conditioning Research* 23 (3): 962-71.

Linnam, V., A. Parkarinen, P. Komi, W. Kraemer, and K. Häkkinen. 2005. "Acute Hormonal Responses to Submaximal and Maximal Heavy Resistance and Explosive Exercises in Men and Women." *Journal of Strength and Conditioning Research* 19 (3): 566-71.

Marquez, C.M., B. Vanaudenaerde, T. Troosters, and N. Wenderoth. 2015. "High-Intensity Interval Training Evokes Larger Serum BDNF Levels Compared With Intense Continuous Exercise." *Journal of Applied Physiology* 119:1363-73.

Masoro, E., and S. Austad. 2011. *Handbook of the Biology of Aging*. 7th ed. London: Elsevier.

McDonald, R. 2019. *Biology of Aging*. 2nd ed. New York: CRC Press.

Medina, J. 2017. *Brain Rules for Aging Well*. Seattle: Pear Press.

Myers, T. 2014. *Anatomy Trains: Myofascial Meridians for Manual and Movement Therapists*. 3rd ed. London: Elsevier.

Pocari, J., C. Bryant, and F. Comana. 2015. *Exercise Physiology*. Philadelphia: F.A. Davis.

Rice, J., and J. Keogh. 2009. "Power Training: Can It Improve Functional Performance in Older Adults? A Systematic Review." *International Journal of Exercise Science* 2 (2): 131-51.

Sayers, S., and K. Gibson. 2010. "A Comparison of High-Speed Power Training and Traditional Slow-Speed Resistance Training in Older Men and Women." *Journal of Strength and Conditioning Research* 24 (12): 3369-80.

Schleip, R. 2015. *Fascia in Sport and Movement*. Edinburgh: Handspring.

Schleip, R. 2017. *Fascial Fitness: How to be Resilient, Elegant, and Dynamic in Everyday Life and Sport*. Chichester, England: Lotus.

Schoenfeld, B. 2016. *Science and Development of Muscle Hypertrophy*. Champaign, IL: Human Kinetics.

Serra, C., S. Bhasin, F. Tangherlini, E. Barton, M. Ganno, A. Zhang, J. Shansky, et al. 2011. "The Role of GH and IGF-1 in Mediating Anabolic Effects of Testosterone on Androgen-Responsive Muscle." *Endocrinology* 152 (1): 193-206.

Szuhany, K., M. Bugatti, and M. Otto. 2015. "A Meta-Analytic Review of the Effects on Brain Derived Neurotrophic Factor." *Journal of Psychiatric Research* 60 (1): 56-64.

Taylor, A., and M. Johnson. 2008. *Physiology of Exercise and Healthy Aging*. Champaign, IL: Human Kinetics.

Taylor, D. 2013. "Physical Activity Is Medicine for Older Adults." *Postgraduate Medical Journal* 90:26-32.

Tosato, M., V. Zamboni, A. Ferrini, and M. Cesari. 2007. "The Aging Process and Potential Interventions to Extend Life Expectancy." *Clinical Interventions in Aging* 2 (3): 401-12.

Voss, M., L. Nagamatsu, T. Liu-Ambrose, and A. Kramer. 2011. "Exercise, Brain and Cognition Across the Life Span." *Journal of Applied Physiology* 111:1505-13.

World Health Organization. "Health Promotion: More Physical Activity." Accessed April 27, 2020. www.who.int/dietphysicalactivity/factsheet_inactivity/en/.

Chapter 3

Berryman, N., L. Bherer, S. Nadeau, L. Lehr, F. Bobeuf, M. Kergoat, T. Vu, and L. Bosquert. 2013. "Executive Functions, Physical Fitness and Mobility in Well-Functioning Older Adults." *Experimental Gerontology* 48:1402-09.

Fragala, M., E. Cadore, S. Dorgo, M. Izquierdo, W. Kraemer, M. Peterson, and E. Ryan. 2019. "Resistance Training for Older Adults: Position Statement From the National Strength and Conditioning Association." *Journal of Strength and Conditioning Research* 33 (8): 2019-52.

Healey, K., D. Hatfield, P. Blanpied, L. Dorfman, and D. Riebe. 2013. "The Effects of Myofascial Release with Foam Rolling on Performance." *Journal of Strength and Conditioning Research* 28 (1): 61-68.

MacDonald, G., D. Button, E. Drinkwater, and D. Behm. 2013a. "Foam Rolling as a Recovery Tool After an Intense Bout of Physical Activity." *Medicine & Science in Sports & Exercise* 46 (1): 131-42.

MacDonald, G., M. Penney, M. Mullaley, A. Cuconato, C. Drake, D. Behm, and D. Button. 2013b. "An Acute Bout of Self-Myofascial Release Increases Range of Motion Without a Subsequent Decrease in Muscle Activation or Force." *Journal of Strength and Conditioning Research* 27 (3): 812-21.

Mauntel, T., M. Clark, and D. Padua. 2014. "Effectiveness of Myofascial Release Therapies on Physical Performance Measurements: A Systematic Review." *Athletic Training & Sports Health Care* 6 (4): 189-96.

Mohr, A., B. Long, and C. Goad. 2014. "Effect of Foam Rolling and Static Stretching on Passive Hip-Flexion Range of Motion." *Journal of Sport Rehabilitation* 23:296-99.

Myers, T. 2014. *Anatomy Trains: Myofascial Meridians for Manual and Movement Therapists*. 3rd ed. London: Elsevier.

Schleip, R. 2015. *Fascia in Sport and Movement*. Edinburgh: Handspring.

Schleip, R. 2017. *Fascial Fitness: How to Be Resilient, Elegant, and Dynamic in Everyday Life and Sport*. Chichester, England: Lotus.

Schmidt, R., and C. Wrisberg. 2004. *Motor Learning and Performance*. 3rd ed. Champaign, IL: Human Kinetics.

Shah, S., and A. Bhalara. 2012. "Myofascial Release." *International Journal of Health Sciences and Research* 2 (2): 69-77.

Chapter 4

Schleip, R. 2017. *Fascial Fitness: How to Be Resilient, Elegant, and Dynamic in Everyday Life and Sport*. Chichester, England: Lotus.

Chapter 5

Baechle, T., and R. Earle. 2008. *Essentials of Strength Training and Conditioning*. 3rd ed. Champaign, IL: Human Kinetics.

Baker, J., M. Bemben, M. Anderson, and D. Bemben. 2006. "Effects of Age on Testosterone Responses to Resistance Exercise and Musculoskeletal Variables in Men." *Journal of Strength and Conditioning Research* 20 (4): 874-81.

Bubbico, A., and L. Kravitz. 2011. "Muscle Hypertrophy: New Insights and Training Recommendations." *IDEA Fitness Journal* 8 (10): 23-26.

Carrol, T., R. Herbert, J. Munn, M. Lee, and S. Gandevia. 2006. "Contralateral Effects of Unilateral Strength Training: Evidence and Possible Mechanisms." *Journal of Applied Physiology* 101 (5): 1514-20.

Church, D., J. Hoffman, G. Mangine, A. Jajtner, J. Townsend, K. Beyer, R. Wang, M. La Monica, D. Fukuda, and J. Stout. 2016. "Comparison of High-intensity vs. High-Volume Resistance Training on the BDNF Response to Exercise." *Journal of Applied Physiology* 121 (16): 123-28.

Cirer-Sastre, R., J. Beltran-Garrido, and F. Corbi. 2017. "Contralateral Effects after Unilateral Strength Training: A Meta-Analysis Comparing Training Loads." *Journal of Sports Science and Medicine* 16 (2): 180-86.

Crewther, C., J. Keogh, J. Cronin, and C. Cook. 2006. "Possible Stimuli for Strength and Power Adaptation: Acute Hormonal Responses." *Sports Medicine* 36 (3): 215-38.

Fragala, M., E. Cadore, S. Dorgo, M. Izquierdo, W. Kraemer, M. Peterson, and E. Ryan. 2019. "Resistance Training for Older Adults: Position Statement From the National Strength and Conditioning Association." *Journal of Strength and Conditioning Research* 33 (8): 2019-52.

Green, L., and D. Gabriel. 2018. "The Cross Education of Strength and Skill Following Unilateral Strength Training in the Upper and Lower Limbs." *Journal of Neurophysiology* 120 (2): 468-79.

Guizelini, P., R. de Aguiar, B. Denadai, F. Caputo, and C. Greco. 2018. "Effect of Resistance Training on Muscle Strength and Rate of Force Development in Healthy Older Adults: A Systematic Review and Meta-Analysis." *Experimental Gerontology* 102 (18): 51-58.

Haff, G., and N. Triplett. 2016. *Essentials of Strength Training and Conditioning*. 4th ed. Champaign, IL: Human Kinetics.

Kraemer, W., and N. Ratamess. 2005. "Hormonal Responses and Adaptations to Resistance Exercise and Training." *Sports Medicine* 35 (4): 339-61.

Kraschnewski, J., C. Sciamanna, J. Poger, L. Rovniak, E. Lehman, A. Cooper, N. Ballentine, and J. Ciccolo. 2016. "Is Strength Training Associated with Mortality Benefits? A 15 Year Cohort Study of US Older Adults." *Preventive Medicine* 87:121.

McDonald, R. 2019. *Biology of Aging*. 2nd ed. New York: CRC Press.

McGill, S. 2010. "Core Training: Evidence Translating to Better Performance and Injury Prevention." *Strength and Conditioning Journal* 22 (3): 33-46.

McGill, S., A. McDermott, and C. Fenwick. 2009. "Comparison of Different Strongman Muscle Activation and Lumbar Spine Motion, Load and Stiffness." *Journal of Strength and Conditioning Research* 23 (4): 1148-61.

Rowe, J.W., and R.L. Kahn. 1998. *Successful Aging*. New York: Pantheon/Random House.

Santana, J.C., F. Vera-Garcia, and S. McGill. 2007. "A Kinetic and Electromyographic Comparison of the Standing Cable Press and Bench Press." *Journal of Strength and Conditioning Research* 21 (4): 1271-79.

Schoenfeld, B. 2010. "The Mechanisms of Muscle Hypertrophy and Their Application to Resistance Training." *Journal of Strength and Conditioning Research* 24 (10): 2857-72.

Schoenfeld, B. 2013. "Potential Mechanisms for a Role of Metabolic Stress in Hypertrophic Adaptations to Resistance Training" *Sports Medicine* 43:179-94.

Schoenfeld, B. 2016. *Science and Development of Muscle Hypertrophy*. Champaign, IL: Human Kinetics.

Spangenburg, E. 2009. "Changes in Muscle Mass with Mechanical Load: Possible Cellular Mechanisms." *Applied Physiology, Nutrition and Metabolism* 34:328-35.

Taylor, A., and M. Johnson. 2008. *Physiology of Exercise and Healthy Aging*. Champaign, IL: Human Kinetics.

U.S. Department of Health and Human Services. 2018. *Physical Activity Guidelines for Americans*. 2nd ed. Washington, DC: U.S. Department of Health and Human Services.

Valls, M., I. Dimauro, A. Brunelli, E. Tranchita, E. Ciminelli, P. Caserotti, G. Duranti, S. Sabatini, A. Parisi, and D. Caporossi. 2014. "Explosive Type of Moderate-Resistance Training Induces Functional, Cardiovascular and Molecular Adaptations in the Elderly." *AGE* 36 (14): 759-72.

Verkhoshansky, Y., and M. Siff. 2009. *Supertraining*. 6th ed. Denver: Supertraining Institute.

Vingren, J., W. Kraemer, N. Ratamess, J. Anderson, J. Volek, and C. Maresh. 2010. "Testosterone Physiology in Resistance Exercise and Training" *Sports Medicine* 40 (12): 1037-53.

Volaklis, K., M. Halle, and C. Meisinger. 2015. "Muscular Strength as a Strong Predictor of Mortality: A Narrative Review." *European Journal of Internal Medicine* 26 (15): 303-10.

Wernbom, M., J. Augustsson, and R. Thomee. 2007. "The Influence of Frequency, Intensity, Volume and Mode of Strength Training on Whole Muscle Cross-Sectional Area in Humans." *Sports Medicine* 37 (3): 225-64.

Zatsiorsky, V., W. Kraemer, and A. Fry. 2021. *Science and Practice of Strength Training.* 3rd ed. Champaign, IL: Human Kinetics.

Chapter 6

Farinatti, P.T., A.A. Geraldes, M.F. Bottaro, M.V. Lima, R.B. Albuquerque, and S.J. Fleck. 2013. "Effects of Different Resistance Training Frequencies on the Muscle Strength and Functional Performance of Active Women Older Than 60 Years." *Journal of Strength and Conditioning Research* 27 (8): 2225-34.

Fragala, M., E. Cadore, S. Dorgo, M. Izquierdo, W. Kraemer, M. Peterson, and E. Ryan. 2019. "Resistance Training for Older Adults: Position Statement From the National Strength and Conditioning Association." *Journal of Strength and Conditioning Research* 33 (8): 2019-52.

Keogh, J., C. Newlands, S. Blewett, A. Payne, and L. Chun-Er. 2010a. "A Kinematic Analysis of a Strongman-Type Event: The Heavy Sled Sprint-Style Pull." *Journal of Strength and Conditioning Research* 24 (11): 3088-97.

Keogh J., A. Payne, B. Anderson, and P. Atkins. 2010b. "A Brief Description of the Biomechanics and Physiology of a Strongman Event: The Tire Flip." *Journal of Strength and Conditioning Research* 24 (3): 1223-28.

McGill, S. 2010. "Core Training: Evidence Translating to Better Performance and Injury Prevention." *Strength and Conditioning Journal* 22 (3): 33-46.

McGill, S., A. McDermott, and C. Fenwick. 2009. "Comparison of Different Strongman Muscle Activation and Lumbar Spine Motion, Load and Stiffness." *Journal of Strength and Conditioning Research* 23 (4): 1148-61.

Winwood, P., J. Keogh, and N. Harris. 2011. "The Strength and Conditioning Practices of Strongman Competitors." *Journal of Strength and Conditioning Research* 25 (11): 3118-28.

Zemke, B., and G. Wright. 2011. "The Use of Strongman Type Implements and Training to Increase Sport Performance in Collegiate Athletes." *Strength and Conditioning Journal* 33:1-7.

Chapter 7

Bryant, C., S. Merrill, and D. Green. 2014. *American Council on Exercise Personal Trainer Manual.* 5th ed. San Diego: American Council on Exercise.

Ciolac, E. 2012. "High-Intensity Interval Training and Hypertension: Maximizing the Benefits of Exercise?" *American Journal of Cardiovascular Disease* 2 (2): 102-10.

Dalleck, L., T. Cuddy, B. Krattenmaker, and D. Green. 2019. "Ace-Sponsored Research: What Are the Acute and Chronic Responses to Reduced-Exertion High-intensity Training?" *CERTIFIED*, May 2019. www.acefitness.org/education-and-resources/professional/certified/may-2019/7267/ace-sponsored-research-what-are-the-acute-and-chronic-responses-to-reduced-exertion-high-intensity-training/.

Elliott, B., P. Herbert, N. Sculthorpe, F. Grace, D. Stratton, and L. Hayes. 2017. "Lifelong Exercise, but Not Short-Term HIIT, Increases GDF11, a Marker of Successful Aging: A Preliminary Investigation." *Physiological Reports* 5 (13): 1-8.

Eston, R. 2012. "Use of Ratings of Perceived Exertion in Sports." *International Journal of Sports Physiology and Performance* 12 (7): 175-82.

Gibala, M., and C. Shulgan 2017. *The One-Minute Workout: Science Shows a Way to Get Fit That's Smarter, Faster, Shorter.* New York: Random House.

Gomes-Neto, M., A. Duraes, H. Correia dos Reis, V. Neves, B. Martinez, and V. Carvalho. 2017. "High-Intensity Interval Training Versus Moderate-Intensity Continuous Training on Exercise Capacity and Quality of Life in Patients with Coronary Artery Disease: A Systematic Review and Meta-Analysis." *European Journal of Preventive Cardiology* 24 (16): 1696-707.

Gries, K., U. Raue, R. Perkins, K. Lavin, B. Overstreet, L. D'Acquisto, B. Graham, et al. 2018. "Cardiovascular and Skeletal Muscle Health with Lifelong Exercise." *Journal of Applied Physiology* 125:1636-45.

Gunnarson, T.P., and J. Bangsbo. 2012. "The 10-20-30 Training Concept Improves Performance and Health Profile in Moderately Trained Runners." *Journal of Applied Physiology* 5 (113): 16-24.

Haff, G., and N. Triplett. 2016. *Essentials of Strength and Conditioning.* 4th ed. Champaign, IL: Human Kinetics.

Hayes, L., P. Herbert, N. Sculthorpe, and F. Grace. 2017. "Exercise Training Improves Free Testosterone in Lifelong Sedentary Aging Men." *Endocrine Connections* 6:306-10.

Kenney, W., J. Wilmore, and D. Costill. 2015. *Physiology of Sport and Exercise*. 6th ed. Champaign, IL: Human Kinetics.

Linnam, V., A. Parkarinen, P. Komi, W. Kraemer, and K. Häkkinen. 2005. "Acute Hormonal Responses to Submaximal and Maximal Heavy Resistance and Explosive Exercises in Men and Women." *Journal of Strength and Conditioning Research* 19 (3): 566-71.

Meckel, Y., D. Nemet, S. Bar-Sela, S. Radom-Aizik, D. Cooper, M. Sagiv, and A. Elliakim. 2011. "Hormonal and Inflammatory Responses to Different Types of Sprint Interval Training." *Journal of Strength and Conditioning Research* 25 (8): 2161-69.

Nilsson, M., and M. Tarnopolsky. 2019. "Mitochondria and Aging—The Role of Exercise as a Countermeasure." *Biology* 40 (8): 1-18.

Robergs, R., and R. Landwehr. 2002. "The Surprising History of the 'HRmax = 220 − age' Equation." *Journal of Exercise Physiology Online* 5 (2). www.asep.org/asep/asep/May2002JEPonline.html.

Salom Huffman, L., D. Wadsworth, J. McDonald, S. Foote, H. Hyatt, and D. Pascoe. 2017. "Effects of a Sprint Interval and Resistance Concurrent Exercise Training Program on Aerobic Capacity of Inactive Adult Women." *Journal of Strength and Conditioning Research* 33 (6): 1640-47.

Schaun, G., S. Pinto, M. Silva, D. Dolinski, and C. Alberton. 2018. "Whole-Body High-Intensity Interval Training Induce Similar Cardiorespiratory Adaptations Compared with Traditional High-Intensity Interval Training and Moderate-Intensity Continuous Training in Healthy Men." *Journal of Strength and Conditioning Research* 32 (10): 2730-42.

Seo, D., S. Lee, N. Kim, K. Ko, B. Rhee, and J. Han. 2016. "Age-Related Changes in Skeletal Muscle Mitochondria: The Role of Exercise." *Integrative Medicine Research* 16 (5): 182-86.

Tabata, I., K. Nishimura, M. Kouzaki, Y. Hirai, F. Ogita, M. Miyachi, and K. Yamamoto. 1996. "Effects of Moderate-Intensity Endurance and High-Intensity Intermittent Training on Anaerobic Capacity and VO2 Max." *Medicine & Science in Sports & Exercise* 28 (10): 1327-30.

Wyckelsma, V., I. Levinger, M. McKenna, L. Formosa, M. Ryan, A. Petersen, M. Anderson, and R. Murphy. 2017. "Preservation of Skeletal Muscle Mitochondria Content in Older Adults: Relationship Between Fiber Type and High Intensity Exercise Training." *Journal of Physiology* 17 (11): 3345-59.

Chapter 8

Brienen, N., A. Timen, J. Wallinga, J. Van Steenbergen, and P. Teunis. 2010. "The Effect of Mask Use on the Spread of Influenza During a Pandemic." *Risk Analysis* 30 (8): 1210-18.

Gleeson, M. 2007. "Immune Function in Sport and Exercise." *Journal of Applied Physiology* 103:693-99.

Haff, G., and N. Triplett. 2016. *Essentials of Strength and Conditioning*. 4th ed. Champaign, IL: Human Kinetics.

Halabchi, F., Z. Ahmadinejad, and M. Selk-Ghaffari. 2020. "COVID-19 Epidemic: Exercise or Not to Exercise; That Is the Question!" *Asian Journal of Sports Medicine* 11 (1): e102630. https://doi.org/10.5812/asjsm.102630.

Hoffman, J. 2014. *Physiological Aspects of Sport Training and Performance*. 2nd ed. Champaign, IL: Human Kinetics.

Peake, J., O. Neubauer, N. Walsh, and R. Simpson. 2017. "Recovery of the Immune System After Exercise." *Journal of Applied Physiology* 122:1077-87.

Simpson, R.J., J.P. Campbell, M. Gleeson, K. Kruger, D.C. Nieman, D.B. Pyne, J.E. Turner, and N.P. Walsh. 2020. "Can Exercise Affect Immune Function to Increase Susceptibility to Infection?" *Exercise Immunology Review* 26:8-22.

Simpson, R.J., and E. Katsanis. 2020. "The Immunological Case for Staying Active During the COVID-19 Pandemic." *Brain, Behavior and Immunity* 87:6-7.

Simpson, R.J., H. Kunz, N. Agha, and R. Graff. 2015. "Exercise and the Regulation of Immune Functions." *Progress in Molecular Biology and Translational Science* 135:355-80.

Verkhoshansky, Y., and M. Siff. 2009. *Supertraining*. 6th ed. Denver: Supertraining Institute.

Wilson, J., P. Marin, M. Rhea, S. Wilson, J. Loenneke, and J. Anderson. 2012. "Concurrent Training: A Meta-Analysis Examining Interference of Aerobic and Resistance Exercises." *Journal of Strength and Conditioning Research* 26 (8): 2293-307.

About the Author

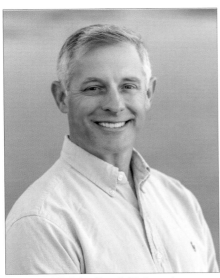

Courtesy of Christine Ekeroth Photography.

Pete McCall is the owner and president of All About Fitness and host of the All About Fitness podcast. He is certified as a personal trainer through the American Council on Exercise (ACE) and the National Academy of Sports Medicine (NASM), and he holds a CSCS (Certified Strength and Conditioning Specialist) certification from the National Strength and Conditioning Association (NSCA). He is the author of *Smarter Workouts: The Science of Exercise Made Simple.*

McCall is a sought-after resource for accurate, in-depth insight on how to get results from exercise. He is frequently quoted as a fitness expert in national publications such as *Wall Street Journal, New York Times, Washington Post, Men's Fitness, Shape,* and *Self.* McCall has more than a decade of experience educating personal trainers around the world, including teaching for both ACE and NASM. He is a master trainer for Core Health & Fitness (the parent company of Nautilus, StairMaster, Star Trac, and Schwinn), a content contributor for 24 Hour Fitness, and an adjunct faculty member in exercise science at both Mesa Community College and San Diego State University. He has delivered wellness education talks for the U.S. Navy (at Naval Air Station North Island), the White House, the World Bank, the International Association of Fire Fighters, and Reebok.

McCall earned his master's of science degree in exercise science and health promotion from the California University of Pennsylvania, and he holds the Fellow in Applied Functional Science credential from the Gray Institute.

McCall is a semiretired rugby player, playing front row forward (all three positions) for Santa Monica Rugby Club, Potomac Athletic Club, and the Boston Irish Wolfhounds, where he was a member of the 2007 men's Division III national championship team. He enjoys mountain biking, obstacle course races, hiking, keeping up with his two children, and coaching youth rugby.

You read the book—now complete the companion CE exam to earn continuing education credit!

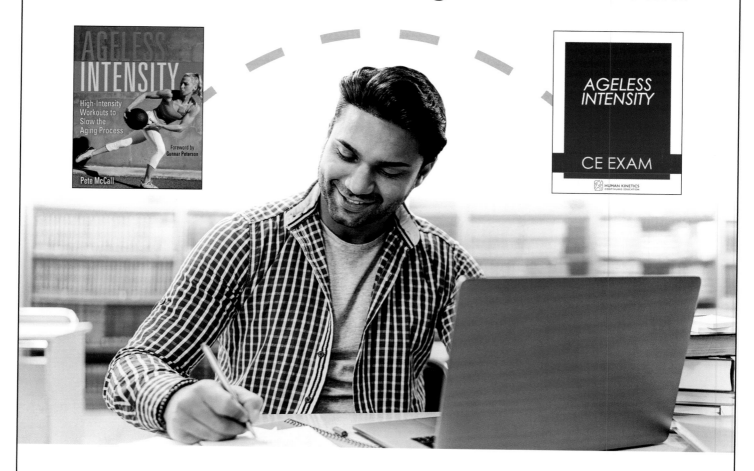

Find and purchase the companion CE exam here:
US.HumanKinetics.com/collections/CE-Exam
Canada.HumanKinetics.com/collections/CE-Exam

50% off the companion CE exam with this code

AI2022

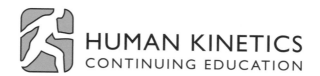